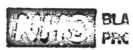 
Prevention and Management
of Hip Fractures

Prevention and Management of Hip Fractures

LIZ ONSLOW MSc, BA (Hons), RN
Southampton University Hospitals NHS Trust

W
WHURR PUBLISHERS
LONDON AND PHILADELPHIA

© 2005 Whurr Publishers Ltd (a subsidiary of John Wiley & Sons, Ltd)
First published 2005
by Whurr Publishers Ltd
The Atrium, Southern Gate, Chichester,
West Sussex, PO19 8SQ, UK
Telephone: (+44) 1243 779777

Email: cs-books@wiley.co.uk
Visit our Home Page on www.wiley.co.uk

British Library Cataloguing in Publication Data

A catalogue record for this book
is available from the British Library.

ISBN 1 86156 501 1

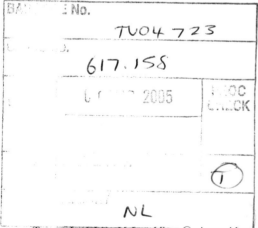
Typeset by Adrian McLaughlin, a@microguides.net
Printed and bound in the UK by TJ International Ltd, Padstow, Cornwall

Contents

Review by orthogeriatric liaison team
A–Z of anaesthesia for hip fracture patients
Traffic light system
Care pathway
Audit
Appendix: The A–Z of anaesthesia for hip fracture patients

Preface

Fractured neck of femur is a condition greatly feared by many elderly people. In my work as a ward sister and specialist nurse I have come to recognize the unique challenges associated with caring for patients with femoral neck fracture. Their journey of care is a complex one, which needs to be well managed from the moment they arrive in the Accident and Emergency department until their discharge from the acute environment, through the rehabilitation process and their eventual discharge. With improved knowledge and a commitment to preventative strategies, we can do much to help reduce the incidence of hip fracture in the future.

The aim of this book is to develop the reader's knowledge and skills in both theory and practice and to encourage the reader to apply this knowledge when caring for people who have fractured their hip. The book emphasizes the importance of collaborative working to promote effective rehabilitation and improve outcomes. I hope that this book will assist nurses and allied health professionals to meet the complex needs of this client group.

Acknowledgements

I am extremely grateful to all the people who have supported me through my own journey towards publication of this book. In particular I would like to thank Edna Dunn, Julia Stanners and Claire Davey, three very special nurses who in their own individual ways have provided the support and encouragement that I have needed and have contributed enormously to the care of older people with hip fracture admitted to our local acute NHS trust hospital.

Thanks also to Dr Lucy White, Consultant Anaesthetist at Southampton University Hospitals NHS Trust, for allowing me to include her 'A to Z of anaesthesia' as an appendix to Chapter 7.

A special thank you to John and Laura, who have coped admirably with being denied access to the family computer and have shared in the highs and lows that have accompanied the writing of this book.

Finally, thank you to all the patients for whom I have been privileged to care. They have assisted me enormously by sharing their 'lived experiences' of coping with a hip fracture, helping me to reflect upon the care that I deliver and seeking out new ways of working that will enhance the care delivery for future patients.

Liz Onslow
Southampton
April 2005

Introduction

This book is written with the intention of providing nurses and allied health professionals with a comprehensive text that can be used when caring for patients with femoral neck fracture, at whatever stage they are at in their journey of care.

People who have sustained a hip fracture are admitted to trauma wards on a background of medical, psychological and/or functional frailty. They face a complex journey of care, with many obstacles to overcome on the journey. The difficulties that they may encounter and the challenges that staff face caring for them have shaped the way that this book is written.

The book takes the reader through the different stages of the patient's journey. It begins with an overview of the epidemiology of hip fracture, anatomy and physiology. It then moves through the assessment process to an extensive review of the factors that need to be considered when caring for the patient with a hip fracture through the various stages of health and social care delivery. These chapters emphasize the importance of using a holistic approach to care and recognizing the skills that each profession brings to optimizing outcomes for this patient group.

Consideration is also given to preventive measures that can be taken to reduce the incidence of hip fracture, and the influence of national policy on shaping services for hip fracture patients. The final chapter explores the current state of hip fracture care and considers implications for the future. This book is designed to be read as a whole, but each chapter will stand alone and can be used to answer specific queries.

Femoral neck fracture is a condition much feared by many older people. Professionals can work collaboratively to reduce the risk of hip fracture or, when injury has occurred, assist individuals as they travel through their journey of care. This book will help professionals to meet the challenge of caring for people who have sustained a hip fracture with confidence and understanding.

CHAPTER ONE

Epidemiology, morbidity and mortality

Femoral neck fracture is a major cause of morbidity and mortality in older people. The costs of this injury not only have an impact on the individuals themselves but also place a considerable strain on an already overstretched health service in general and orthopaedic departments in particular. It is estimated that more than one fifth of the available orthopaedic beds in UK hospitals are occupied by hip fracture patients (RCP/BTS 1999). In the UK approximately 70 000 people each year fracture their hip after a fall (Torgerson and Dolan 1998), and this figure is predicted to rise.

Any strategies to prevent the predicted rise in hip fractures must be based on a sound knowledge of the aetiopathology of hip fracture, and the purpose of this chapter is to assist the reader in understanding the complex area of risk factors for hip fracture and the reasons for its high morbidity and mortality rates. There are two categories of hip fracture: high-energy fractures which typically occur in younger adults and low-energy fractures which occur in older people. In this chapter, the focus is on low-energy hip fractures.

Femoral neck fracture is an extremely serious injury, with a reported mortality rate of 13–27% (Egol and Koval 2002, Goldacre et al. 2002). The risk of hip fracture rises exponentially with age, with a woman aged 50 years having a 15% chance of sustaining a hip fracture during her lifetime. At the age of 90, one in three women will have sustained a fractured neck of femur (Ellis 2003). The number of people over the age of 65 years is rising, and with this increase in the ageing population a rise in the number of hip fractures can also be predicted. This is associated not only with the ageing population but also with the increase in the rate of hip fracture (number of people per head of population). The number of hip fractures worldwide is expected to rise from 1.7 million in 1990 to approximately 6.3 million in 2050 (Aharanoff et al. 1997).

Worldwide predictions for hip fracture have highlighted specific areas for concern. In the 1960s, there were notable variations in hip fracture incidence, with the highest incidence in northern Europe and North America. However, results from the Asian Osteoporosis Study confirmed that the incidence of hip fracture rates in Hong Kong and Singapore were

1

approaching those observed in white Americans, and although rates in Malaysia and Thailand were much lower, they are likely to increase with urbanization and ageing. It is estimated that by 2050 more than 50% of all hip fractures will occur in Asia (Lau et al. 2001).

In England and Wales the number of hip fractures based on population growth alone is estimated to rise to approximately 60 000 cases per year by 2016. Estimates based on increasing rates of hip fracture could almost double this number to 117 000 cases (Audit Commission 1995).

It has been suggested that under current patterns of care, the higher estimate would require extra beds and other resources equivalent to eight District General Hospitals by 2015 (Audit Commission 1995). Preventive strategies that are being followed to reduce the incidence of hip fractures are discussed in the next two chapters, but it is necessary at this early stage to recognize that the challenge of the hip fracture epidemic is one that requires urgent and continued attention. In rising to the challenge, medical staff, nurses and allied health professionals must recognize the complexity of factors in hip fracture risk (Allolio 1999). Some of these factors are related to skeletal factors, others to falls, and there are other more complex factors that sit between the two (Fig. 1.1, Table 1.1).

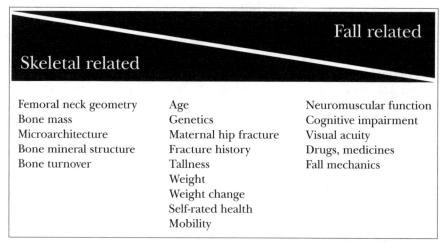

Figure 1.1 Risk factors for hip fracture. (Source: Bandolier 1998). Reprinted with kind permission of Bandolier@pru.ox.ac.uk

Risk factors relating to skeletal factors and falls are considered in separate chapters; in this chapter the focus is on the complex factors that are intermediate between the two. In considering these, it must be acknowledged that not all factors considered in the aetiopathology of hip fracture can be examined in this chapter, and some theories are still controversial.

Table 1.1 Risk factors for hip fracture in women

Risk factor	Comment
Skeletal-related risk factors	
Femoral neck geometry	Longer hip axis (trochanter to pelvic rim) increases risk of fractured neck of femur
Microarchitecture	Bone strength is associated with increased risk, and can be measured with broadband ultrasound attenuation. Risk increased about 7-fold in women above versus below median heel ultrasound measures
Mineral structure	Fluoride may increase bone strength
Bone turnover	Biochemical markers of increased bone turnover may be related to increased risk
Fall-related risk factors	
Neuromuscular function	Inability to rise from chair unaided five times, or on feet for fewer than 4 hours a day, inability to heel-to-toe walk all associated with increased risk
Cognitive impairment	Poor mental health is a risk factor
Medications and drugs	Sedative use, longacting benzodiazepines increase risk. Caffeine consumption increases risk
Fall mechanics	Fall on side highly increases risk
Complex risk factors	
Age	Most hip fractures occur after 75 years
Genetic background	Maternal hip fracture increases risk. Some genetic markers are being studied which might be useful predictors of increased risk
Body size	Being tall at a young age, being thin, or losing more than 10% of body weight since age 25 all increase the risk, while gaining weight may reduce risk
Physical activity	High levels of physical activity, especially walking, are associated with reduced risk of fracture

Source Bandolier 1998. Risk factors for hip fracture in women). Reproduced with kind permission from Bandolier@pru.ox.ac.uk

The aim in discussing a selection of factors is to stimulate the interest of the reader and encourage further exploration of the subject.

Hip fracture in older people usually occurs as a result of a fall laterally on to the hip with a failure of protective reflexes and a lack of absorption of energy by local soft tissue. This is often compounded by a reduction in bone strength. As previously mentioned, the incidence of hip fracture is closely related to age. Changes in vestibular function, the musculoskeletal system and vision all contribute to deterioration in normal postural stability which contributes to the risk and type of falls (Berge et al. 1994). Bone loss usually increases with ageing, and this affects bone strength. These factors are further explored in Chapters 2 and 3.

Sex and race

Differences in risk factors for hip fracture are related to sex and race, with white women having the highest risk. Approximately 17% of 65-year-old white women and 9% of white men can expect to sustain a hip fracture by the age of 90. For black women and men the figures are 5% and 3% respectively (Barnett et al. 1999). For white women, the higher risk of hip fracture is related to their increased propensity to fall and higher levels of bone loss associated with menopause (McCosty and Coopman 1993, Melton 1993). Among men the risk is attributed to testosterone deficiency (Grisso et al. 1991, Hemenway et al. 1994). Changes in bone geometry that compensate for age-related reductions in bone strength have also been suggested as contributing to the differences in hip fracture risk between men and women (Mow and Hayes 1997).

Fracture rates are higher in whites than in blacks, with risk rates for Hispanics and Asians being intermediate between these two. There is an indication that these rates are attributable to differences in bone mass and hip geometry (Chin et al. 1997, Theobold et al. 1998), although this is not conclusive. The increased rate of hip fracture in Asia is linked to urbanization, ageing and the adoption of Western lifestyle factors such a low dietary calcium intake, a sedentary lifestyle, cigarette smoking and increased alcohol consumption, all of which are linked to increased risk of osteoporosis (Lau et al. 2001).

Residential factors

Studies relating to urban versus rural community dwellers are conflicting, although they largely report a higher incidence of hip fracture risk in urban dwellers (Baudoin et al. 1993, Madhok et al. 1993). However, these findings must be treated with caution as they may be a reflection of better reporting from urban areas. Other studies challenge these findings, with some indicating an increase in risk among rural dwellers and others identifying no urban–rural differences (Dilsen et al. 1993, Luthje et al. 1995).

Living in an institutional setting such as a nursing home or rest home is also reported to have an impact on predicted risk for hip fracture. With the age and sex adjustments taken into consideration, the incidence of hip fracture is reported to be 10.5–15 times higher than for those living in private homes (Ooms et al. 1993, Butler et al. 1996). These figures are perhaps not surprising when one considers the physical frailty and cognitive decline that is apparent in many nursing and rest home residents. When factors such as these are taken into account along with sex and age, living in an institution is not the prime risk factor. Hip fracture in these circumstances is associated with other risk factors such as propensity to fall and the poorer health status of individuals living in institutional care (Cummings 1996).

Anthropometric factors

Anthropometric factors and their influence on occurrence of hip fracture have been highlighted in many studies. There is, for example, a correlation between above-average height and the subsequent risk of hip fracture (Center et al. 1998, Lau et al. 2001). Explanations include the influence that height might have on the geometrical proportions of the hip (Nakamura et al. 1994) and the force associated with falling that might be increased as a result of height (Hayes et al. 1993). However, although these studies highlight a positive correlation between height and risk of hip fracture, other studies have reported opposite findings (Huopio et al. 2000). Maternal height and a slow rate of growth in childhood are considered to be major determinants of subsequent hip fracture in later life, but the underlying reason for reduced childhood growth rate is still not established (Cooper et al. 2001).

Some studies report lower body weight as an independent predictor of hip fracture (McGrother et al. 2002). Low body weight is also associated with low bone mineral density, which might help explain the high risk of hip fracture in low-weight individuals. Moreover, low body weight is also known to be an indicator of poor health and frailty (Dargent-Molina et al. 2000) and these factors will also contribute to the high risk of hip fracture.

Bone geometry

Studies relating to upper femoral bone geometry including hip axis length, width of the femoral neck and femoral neck angle provide us with another possible important predictor of future hip fracture risk. A number of studies demonstrate that hip axis length is positively correlated with increased hip fracture risk (Karlsson et al. 1996, Gnudi et al. 1999). The torsional strain that occurs on a loaded femur, causing it to break at the femoral neck (its weakest point), has also been pointed out as a factor in bone geometry that may increase the risk of hip fracture: however, many studies relating to pelvic bone geometry have produced conflicting results, particularly in relation to the angle of the femoral shaft (Michelloti and Clark 1999, Alonso et al. 2000).

Gynaecological and familial risk factors

Bone turnover is known to become altered during pregnancy and lactation (Sowers 1996, Holunberg-Martilla and Sievanen 1999). Lactation appears to provide protection against hip fracture risk, with evidence to suggest that in women who breast fed for up to 12 months, irrespective of age, there was protection against hip fracture, although there is uncertainty about the net long-term effect of parity and lactation (Michaelson et al. 2001). A reduced risk of hip fracture is related to later age at menopause, although postmenopausal women who have high serum concentrations of sex hormone globulin and undetectable serum oestradiol concentrations appear to have an increased risk of hip fractures (Cummings et al. 1998). Familial factors and the increased risk of hip fracture have also been reported, with those who have a maternal history of hip fracture being at greatest risk (Fox et al. 1998).

Environmental factors

Environmental risk factors other than falls have been considered in relation to hip fracture risk, but research indicates that the relationship between these and hip fracture is unclear (Parker et al. 1996, Clemson et al. 1996). There is conflicting evidence about seasonal weather variations (Parker et al. 1996, Chesser et al. 2002). Other studies indicate that there are time variations in the incidence of hip fracture. Older adults are most likely to fracture a hip in the morning between the hours of 9 a.m. and noon. It has been argued that this may be because of drug-induced factors such as dizziness caused by hypotensive medications, or activities of daily living that are related to the morning (Parker et al. 1996). The relationship between certain medications and risk of falls and subsequent hip fracture is explored in greater depth in Chapter 3, which covers the incidence, prevention and management of falls.

Lifestyle factors

Several lifestyle factors have also been considered as antecedents for hip fracture. Physical activity, including simple tasks such as doing the daily chores and climbing stairs, have been demonstrated to have a protective effect against hip fracture; the converse is also true in relation to those individuals who are inactive (Gregg et al. 2000, Kujala et al. 2000).

Tobacco smoking has been identified as an independent risk factor for hip fracture in men and women (Hoidrup et al. 2000, Vestergaard and Mosekilde 2003), with the suggestion that relative risk decreases after smoking cessation (Baron et al. 2001). However, some studies indicate that although stopping smoking may be beneficial in reducing hip fracture risk, some of the adverse effects are irreversible (Forsen et al. 1998, Hoidrup et al. 2000).

The biological effects that may influence the risk of a hip fracture as a result of smoking are primarily related to osteoporosis: for example, the adverse effect on bone strength due to the toxic influence of nicotine and non-nicotine components of cigarette smoke on bone cells (Fang et al. 1991). Bone strength may also be indirectly affected through increased metabolism or decreased production of oestrogen and decreased calcium absorption. Some mechanisms that are unrelated to osteoporosis may also influence the risk of hip fracture, such as poor physical performance and balance due to adverse effects on peripheral vascular and neurovascular deterioration caused by cigarette smoking. There is also a suggestion that smoking may affect hip fracture risk through different biological mechanisms in men and women (Hoidrup et al. 2000).

The association between alcohol consumption and hip fracture remains unclear, although there is some indication that moderate alcohol intake appears to help maintain bone density in postmenopausal women (Baron et al. 2001). It has been suggested that this may be related to increased oestrogen levels in moderate drinkers. For people who drink heavily, the risk of hip fracture is increased. This is probably because any benefits gained by the increase in bone density relating to increased oestrogen levels in moderate drinkers will be offset in heavy drinkers by the higher risk of falls.

Results from studies on the role of fluorine as an antecedent for hip fracture risk remain inconsistent, with some studies suggesting a positive association between the concentration of fluoride in water and incidence of hip fracture (Jacquim-Gadda et al. 1995). More recent studies refute these findings and argue that there is no association (Hallier et al. 2000, Phipps et al. 2000). The role of dietary calcium has also been studied, with equivocal results, although there is sufficient evidence to support the combined administration of oral vitamin D and calcium in elderly people who are at high risk of hip fracture (Gillespie et al. 2004). This is further explored in Chapter 2, which focuses on osteoporosis.

In identifying some of the antecedents for hip fracture risk, it has become apparent that the prevention and management of hip fractures provides us with enormous challenges in terms of further research, health education, improving clinical practice and planning for future service provision. For individual patients, a number of contributory factors may increase their risk of hip fracture and these must be taken into account. For most patients who sustain this injury, however, the precipitating event is a low-impact fall on to the hip.

Mortality and morbidity

As a consequence of the fall and the subsequent hip fracture, the patient begins a journey of care. For many patients, the outcomes are good and they will recover well, returning to their previous homes. Outcomes for other patients in terms of morbidity and mortality will not be so positive, and it is now important to consider why many patients who sustain this injury 'come into the world under the brim of the pelvis and go out through the neck of the femur' (De Lees 1977, cited in Anwar 1999).

Before any attempt is made to consider mortality rates associated with hip fracture, it is necessary to ascertain whether the reported rates are exactly as they seem. This is a difficult question to answer. Concerns have been raised regarding the under-reporting of hip fracture as a cause of death, with the suggestion that hip fractures may not be recorded on death certificates even when death occurs soon after the fracture (Goldacre et al. 2002). Other factors may also have an impact on data presented in hip fracture mortality studies, and it is clearly important to understand these factors if we are attempting to scrutinize the data presented. An illustration of this is the mortality rates in men, which are known to be higher than in women. Studies that have a high proportion of men in their sample are likely to show higher inpatient mortality rates (US Congress 1994). Inpatient mortality rates will also be affected by the average length of hospital stay, which in many areas has been decreasing over recent years. A low inpatient mortality rate could be misleading, when we consider that some patients who might have died in hospital if hospital stays were longer will now die at home, or in a nursing home, after their discharge. Conversely, there may be a number of patients awaiting nursing home placement who remain on an acute ward while awaiting transfer, despite being medically fit to be discharged to a residential facility. Some of these patients will die in hospital while awaiting placement, and this will be reflected in an increased inpatient mortality rate. It is therefore important to recognize these factors and to measure mortality rates for hip fracture beyond the acute hospital environment.

The presentation of comparative mortality data can also be misleading if the issue of case mix is not addressed, with factors that may have an impact on prognosis being taken into account – for example, age, sex, type of fracture and pre-existing conditions such as stroke, dementia or cardiac failure (Bedford 1996). Despite the highlighted difficulties associated with the collection, presentation and interpretation of hip fracture mortality data, a great deal of evidence has accumulated which demonstrates the persistently higher mortality rates in hip fracture patients than in the general population of a comparable age, with these increased rates continuing for many months after injury (Heikkinen et al. 2001, Goldacre et al. 2002).

As previously suggested, mortality rates are higher in men than in women even when age, number and type of other diagnoses, and postoperative complications are taken into consideration (Walker et al. 1999, Balasegaram et al. 2001). Racial differences have also been identified in some studies, with mortality rates being higher for white men than for black men and lower for white women than for black women (US Congress 1994). Mortality rates are also higher in patients over 80 years of age (Walker et al. 1999), although one recent study has demonstrated that hip fracture is not associated with significant excess mortality among patients older than age 85 (Richmond et al. 2003).

Reasons for the higher mortality rates in hip fracture patients are not well known. They may be a consequence of the continuing sequelae of the hip fracture itself, or attributable to the fact that people who sustain a hip fracture may be more frail and ill than the general population of a similar age. Predictors of hip fracture mortality appear to give support to this second hypothesis. Many hip fracture patients have at least one co-morbidity common in old age, and co-morbidities such as congestive heart failure, chronic obstructive pulmonary disease and angina are known to increase the risk of mortality (Forsen et al. 1998). Other predictors for increased risk of mortality include poor pre-fracture function, poor baseline mental status and delirium (Fitzpatrick et al. 2001, Richmond et al. 2003). It is not uncommon for hip fracture patients to present with more than one co-morbidity, and these factors will contribute significantly to anaesthetic risk and the possibility of postoperative complications which, if not identified early and managed appropriately, will have a considerable impact on postoperative mortality.

The above-mentioned factors provide us with a persuasive argument to support the development and implementation of good orthogeriatric liaison services, and it has been suggested that outcomes for hip fracture patients are improved in areas where these services exist (Audit Commission 1995, 2000, SIGN 2002). Models of orthogeriatric liaison and the impact that they can have in terms of patient care and outcomes are discussed in Chapter 8.

Numerous studies relating to the timing of surgery support surgical fixation of the hip within 24 hours of injury in medically fit patients if 1-year survival rates are to be improved (Grimes et al. 2002, Casaletto and Gatt 2004). Factors that contribute to higher mortality rates in patients whose surgery is delayed are primarily linked to complications associated with bed rest and lack of mobility, such as atelectasis, hypostatic pneumonia and pulmonary embolism. Hip fracture patients are at significant risk of developing thromboembolic complications, with one study demonstrating that 40–80% develop a deep-vein thrombosis, 10–30% a proximal vein thrombosis and 1–10% a fatal pulmonary embolism if prophylactic measures are not undertaken (Todd et al. 1995).

Clearly, thromboembolic prophylaxis is of paramount importance for this vulnerable group of patients if mortality rates are to be improved. Thromboembolic protocols and their implementation should be a cornerstone of good practice in hip fracture care. Early mobilization also contributes significantly to improved outcomes, and it is factors such as these that make the timing of surgery so crucial to improving survival rates for medically fit patients. Delaying surgery for up to 72 hours does not in itself appear to be associated with an increase in mortality in those patients who have concomitant medical conditions that require stabilization, and it is suggested that in these situations it makes sense to optimize medical problems that are likely to lead to postoperative complications (Audit Commission 1995, 2000, Grimes et al. 2002).

Although there are some contributory factors relating to increased mortality rates over which we have no control, such as age and significant co-morbidities, there are areas in which practitioners can work collaboratively to improve survival rates in those patients who are considered to be medically fit for surgery: for example, the implementation and maintenance of a robust thromboembolic policy and ensuring that surgery is performed within 24 hours of injury. These important factors are discussed in Chapters 6 and 7.

In survivors of hip fracture surgery the primary goal of any rehabilitation programme is to reduce disability and maximize function to enable the person to return to their prefracture home. Evidence does, however, suggest that for many hip fracture patients there is some decline in function (Hall et al. 2000, Rosell and Parker 2003) and in some circumstances this may require an increased level of residential or nursing home care. As with the incidence of mortality, there are several variables that may have an impact upon functional outcomes in hip fracture patients, and it is necessary to understand these if we are to develop effective rehabilitation programmes that address the unique needs of individual patients.

Admission functional status has been identified as the key predictor in functional change for patients with femoral neck fracture (Kelly et al. 2000, Hannan et al. 2001). There is a general consensus in the research literature that a patient's ambulatory status will drop one grade after a hip fracture. For example, a person who previously walked unaided may require a stick, and a person who previously used a walking frame may be limited to transfers only. Obviously these factors will have an impact on other aspects of life: a person who has previously walked with a frame and lived alone at home, but can now only transfer with assistance, may no longer be able to live at home and may require admission to institutional care. Other factors relating to functional outcome after hip fracture include age, pain, co-morbidity, level of social support, socioeconomic status and perceived health and quality of life (Magaziner et al. 2000, Shah et al. 2001).

It is generally accepted that patients who return to living in the community after their hip fracture have the best outcomes. However, when we consider the quality of life as perceived by individuals, the reality can appear somewhat different. It is suggested that a decline in ambulatory status and ability to self care has a greater impact on those living at home than on those living in institutional care. The reduced social and functional independence that some individuals experience on returning to the community is reflected in the diminished quality of life perceived by them (Hall et al. 2000, Salkeld et al. 2000). Returning home will be a very different experience for an individual who may now be dependent upon carers to assist with personal hygiene needs and other daily living activities. Although they recognize that help may be necessary, it will take a period of adjustment to cope with 'strangers' entering their home, with some people feeling that their privacy has been invaded because of these 'strangers'. People who have led a relatively active life until their accident can feel isolated because they are no longer able to go outside alone and may not have anybody to support them with activities that they previously took for granted. For some individuals, social isolation may also result in depression.

Despite difficulties associated with returning home after a fractured hip, and in many circumstances with an accompanying functional and ambulatory decline, the single most important threat for many older people who fracture their hip seems to be the loss of independence, dignity and possessions that accompanies the move from living in their own homes to living in a nursing home. In the study undertaken by Salkeld et al. (2000),

80% of respondents expressed a preference for death rather than a 'bad' hip fracture that would result in admission to a nursing home.

Studies such as those mentioned above should at the very least lead us to examine and reflect on the delivery of rehabilitation programmes for patients who have had a hip fracture. As previously suggested, there is a need to ensure that such programmes focus on the uniqueness of individuals. To ensure that this happens, patients must be actively involved in decisions regarding future plans, and practitioners must ensure that optimizing a person's ability to live independently and to participate in social and other aspects of life are encapsulated in any rehabilitation programme, thus ensuring that enhancing patients' functional mobility and activities are not the only aspects of delivering effective, person-centred rehabilitation. The importance of these factors is highlighted in case studies presented and discussed in Chapter 9.

Health care professionals must also be aware of other factors that may influence the person's successful transition through recovery after hip fracture. Factors that might be described as inhibitory include physical pain and discomfort; dependency; loss of control; impatience and fear of falling; mobility precautions necessary to prevent dislocation of a prosthetic hip, such as avoidance of bending and twisting; or mobility devices which, although important to assist patients, could be viewed as stigmatizing because they reflect a loss of independence (Robinson 1999). Assisting patients to adapt to these inhibitory factors will help to promote their recovery.

The primary predictor for admission to institutional care following hip fracture is a poor baseline mental status (Steiner et al. 1997, Aguero-Torres et al. 1998). Studies of patients with cognitive impairment are limited, however, because recruitment of cognitively impaired patients with hip fracture to trials is difficult for ethical and practical reasons (Quereshi and Seymour 2003). The studies that have been undertaken suggest that patients with mild to moderate dementia can benefit from specialized rehabilitation after hip fracture (Huusko et al. 2000, Beloosesky et al. 2001) and it is therefore important that, as suggested above, we target rehabilitation programmes to meet individual needs.

There is a growing body of knowledge about the aetiopathology, mortality and morbidity of hip fracture in older people. It is essential to use that knowledge to inform our practice when caring for this particularly vulnerable group of patients if we are going to improve outcomes in terms of survival and function. The predicted rise in the number of hip fractures by the year 2050 is frightening, and the associated economic costs will be enormous. The costs for the treatment of hip fractures in the UK are estimated at £5 million pounds a day, an annual cost of approximately £1.7 billion (Torgerson et al. 2000).

The economic burden is compounded by the cost in terms of human suffering for individuals who sustain a hip fracture, many of whom – if they survive – will suffer a decline in ambulatory status and in their ability to undertake activities of daily living that they may previously have taken for granted. It is perhaps not surprising that hip fracture, and its effect on their perceived quality of life, is so greatly feared by older people.

In focusing on high mortality rates and poor outcomes for survivors of hip fracture, the author may appear to be guilty of perpetuating the negativity that is all too pervasive in hip fracture care. I hope, however, that examining these issues has conveyed an underlying message to the reader. This message is that we need to examine all aspects of our practice in terms of approaches to care delivery for this particularly vulnerable group of patients. In increasing our knowledge of the factors highlighted in this opening chapter, health professionals can work towards challenging the status quo and promoting effective care for their patients. Questions have been raised regarding the opportunities that are being lost in relation to the prevention of hip fractures in older people. As we move through the next two chapters, it will become apparent that a great deal can be done to prevent hip fracture by preventing falls and better management of osteoporosis, and it is clearly important that we work together in order to ensure that we find ways to avoid missing opportunities to prevent significant numbers of fractures in the future.

CHAPTER TWO

Osteoporosis

In the previous chapter, attention was drawn to the complexity of factors contributing to hip fracture risk. As suggested there, some of these factors are skeletal related, and the purpose of this chapter is to consider the role of osteoporosis in the aetiology of fragility fractures in general, with a particular focus on hip fracture.

Osteoporosis has been defined as 'a skeletal disorder characterized by compromised bone strength predisposing a person to an increased risk of fracture. Bone strength primarily reflects the integration of bone density and bone quality' (AMA 2001) (Fig. 2.1).

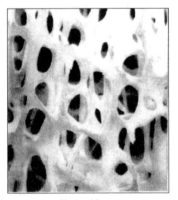
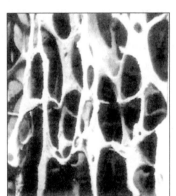

Normal bone   Osteoporosis

Figure 2.1 Normal and osteoporotic bone. (Source: National Osteoporosis Foundation.)

The clinical consequence of osteoporosis is a fracture, which involves the factors: bone fragility, the fall and the impact of the fall. Most people do not know they have a problem with bone fragility until they sustain a fracture. Osteoporosis affects 1 in 3 women and 1 in 12 men over the age of 50 in the UK. It is important to remember that osteoporosis can be prevented and treated, and by doing so the risk of hip fracture can be significantly reduced.

Epidemiology

Osteoporosis is a common condition in the over 50s, causing 310 000 fractures a year in the UK and costing an estimated £1.7 billion (Torgerson et al. 2001). Osteoporotic fractures are usually of the forearm, spine or hip, but may occur at other sites. They are usually described as low-trauma fractures, have a higher incidence in women and an increased incidence with age, and occur at sites of high trabecular bone content.

There is a significant cost to individuals, with a reported 20% excess mortality in the year following hip and vertebral fractures. As suggested in the previous chapter there is also a significant decline in ambulatory status and ability to self care following a hip fracture. Multiple vertebral fractures cause loss of height, kyphosis and severe and chronic back pain, reduced ability to cope with the activities of daily living and poor mood (Scott-Russell et al. 2003).

The absolute lifetime risk of fractures at age 50 in the UK is 53.2% for women and 20.7% for men (van Staa et al. 2001) The fracture rate increases with age, and this is thought to be a consequence of lower bone density and tendency to fall. There is a racial variation, with lower fracture rates in black populations than in white or Asian populations. A geographic variation also exists within countries, perhaps suggesting an environmental aspect (Woolf and Pfleger 2003).

Osteoporotic fractures are already a major public health problem, and with rising life expectancy are going to become more so in the future.

Change in bone mass through life

There is a steady growth of bone mass from birth up to puberty, when a large increase in bone mass occurs in both sexes. Bone mass continues to increase until the mid to late 20s, when it reaches its peak. It then levels out, and begins to decrease after the age of 40 (see Fig. 2.2).

The accumulation of bone mass from infancy to post-puberty involves interrelated actions of genetic, endocrine (hormone), mechanical (exercise) and nutritional factors, and can be influenced by environmental factors. It has been shown that those who undertake more weight-bearing exercise and have a good nutritional intake can achieve a higher peak bone mass (Bonjour et al. 2003). Peak bone mass is an important determinant of fragility fractures in later life, as a 10% increase in peak bone mass will result in a 50% reduction in fractures in later years. In women a greater percentage of bone loss occurs around the menopause.

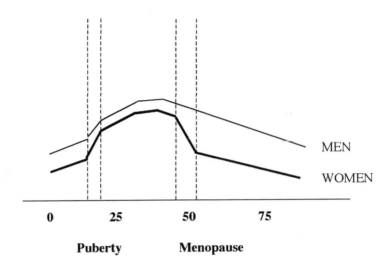

Figure 2.2 Peak bone mass.

Bone remodelling

There are two types of bone:

- **Cortical bone** is compact and makes up around 80% of the skeleton; it is found on the outer shafts of long bone and the surface of flat bones.
- **Trabecular bone** is found at the end of long bones and makes up the inside of flat bones; this has an open woven structure and better nutrient supply.

Bone is made up of an extracellular collagenous matrix and renews itself throughout life: old bone is removed and new bone is laid down. This enables growth and repair to occur, and also enables the bone to respond to any changes in physical stress placed upon it. This renewal process occurs through the bone remodelling cycle.

Bone remodelling is a complex process and results from the interaction of the mechanical stresses placed on the body, hormones and locally produced cytokines, prostaglandins and growth factors. Three types of bone cells are involved in the process:

- **osteocytes**, which are embedded in the bone and appear to have a function in starting the bone remodelling process
- **osteoclasts**, which break down bone
- **osteoblasts**, which build new bone.

The cycle begins with a chemical message from the osteocyte, which attracts osteoclasts to the area of bone to be remodelled. The osteoclasts dissolve the bone by secreting acid and enzymes on to it, breaking down the mineral within the bone, which is washed into the blood stream. The matrix of the bone then breaks down, leading to the formation of a cavity. Once the cavity has been hollowed out, the osteoclast cells move away. Then osteoblasts move into the area and synthesize a substance called osteoid which eventually becomes mineralized bone tissue (see Fig. 2.3).

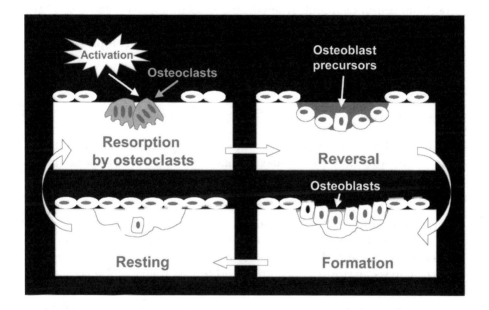

Figure 2.3 Bone remodelling cycle.

Bone remodelling occurs more frequently in areas of trabecular bone, because of its better blood and nutritional supply and its higher surface area compared with cortical bone.

In childhood and adolescence there is a growth in height and density, where the osteoblast cells lay down more bone at each remodelling cycle, resulting in bone growth. By the end of the fourth decade the bone remodelling process occurs more frequently, resulting in a larger number of cavities in the bone at any one time. The osteoblasts are unable to keep up with the osteoclasts, and are therefore unable to completely fill the cavities at each cycle, which results in a net loss of bone.

Osteoporosis

There are two basic mechanisms of bone loss. In terms of amount of bone lost the more important is **bone turnover rate,** which increases the number of bone remodelling units. The other mechanism is **remodelling imbalance**, where the amount of bone formed within individual bone remodelling units is less than it should be. Menopausal bone loss is associated with both these factors. It appears to be a direct consequence of oestrogen deficiency, as it shows a close relationship with oestrogen withdrawal and responds rapidly when oestrogen is replaced (Compston 1994). The bone loss associated with old age appears to be an effect of the remodelling imbalance, where each remodelling cavity is incompletely filled, resulting in a net loss of bone.

Bone quality

The quality of bone must also be considered alongside the density of bone. Bone density probably contributes around 50% of a person's bone fragility fracture risk; the bone quality may explain the remainder. Bone quality could be said to consist of:

- the material of bone (collagen, degree of mineralization)
- architectural factors (thinning of trabecular struts, loss of connectivity between struts and the disappearance of horizontal struts, the loss of cortical mass, periosteal apposition and the geometry of the bone structure itself)
- mechanical characteristics (microdamage accumulation, stiffness, strength, bone size).

The concept of bone quality is currently not completely understood, and certainly cannot be measured as bone density can.

Risk factors

Continuing research and evaluation has established clinical risk factors (Table 2.1) for both osteoporosis and fracture, which are said to be different, but overlapping (AMA 2001).

It is difficult to evaluate the risk factors for osteoporosis, for a number of reasons. One is that the diagnosis of low bone density has different significance at different ages (Kanis et al. 2001), which affects the weighting of the risk factors. The significance of risk factors also varies according to the use being made of them; for example, targeting bone density scans,

Table 2.1 Risk factors for osteoporosis and fracture

Risk factors with the strongest evidence

Age
Gender
Low body weight
Previous fracture
Glucocorticoid use

Risk factors with strong evidence, and also conditions that occur rarely in the population

Family history
Oestrogen/testosterone hormone deficiency
Thyroid and parathyroid disease
Immunosuppressants
Malabsorption disease
Chronic anticonvulsant therapy

Risk factors for which the evidence is less strong

Smoking
Excess alcohol
Diet
Exercise

making treatment decisions or giving advice to encourage an individual to make lifestyle changes.

The risk factors in Table 2.1 with the strongest evidence have been well evaluated, with an acceptance that the risk factor is independent of other factors. They are also relevant across a wide age range. Increasing age, female gender and white and Asian race are well-accepted risk factors, along with low body weight (a body mass index of 19 or less). A number of authors have demonstrated fragility fractures (that is, a fall from head height or less) as independent risk factor for further fracture. Oral corticosteroid therapy is a well-validated risk factor. van Staa et al. (2002a) undertook a meta-analysis and found that higher daily doses of oral corticosteroids and length of time on oral steroids both increased the risk; a higher fracture rate was seen within 3–6 months. No dose of oral steroid therapy was found to be safe.

The effect of glucocorticoids on bone mineral density is dependent on dose, duration and steroid type. The overall affects of glucocorticoids are described by Lane (2001) as impaired bone formation with unchanged or enhanced bone resorption. This suppression of bone formation is the most important effect of the glucocorticoids and is caused by several mechanisms. There are glucocorticoid receptors in most types of cells, including bone cells. Glucocorticoids affect the activity of osteoblast lineage and other cells within bone and adjust the reproduction of the genes responsible for matrix constituents such as collagen and osteocalcin. Further, they are thought to influence the activity of locally acting factors that affect osteoblasts, such as cytokine and growth factors (RCP 2002).

The loss of bone mineral density is greatest within the first few months of steroid therapy, and women and men who take steroids have a higher risk of fractures over and above the effect of low bone mineral density. The guidelines for treatment is a T-score of −1.5 or less, and those over the age of 65 or with a previous fragility fracture should start treatment, ideally with a bisphosphonate, at the time they start their steroid therapy (see Fig. 2.4) (RCP 2002).

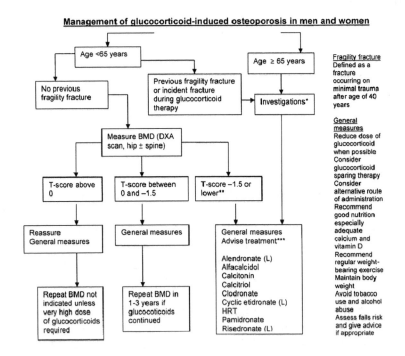

Figure 2.4 Management of men and women with glucocorticoid-induced osteoporosis. Reproduced with kind permission of the Royal College of Physicians.

The effect of inhaled corticosteroids has important implications, as these drugs are widely used by young people. The meta-analysis by van Staa et al. (2002a) found that users of inhaled corticosteroids had an increased fracture rate, but commented that this was related to underlying respiratory disease. Richy et al. (2003) found there was an effect of inhaled corticosteroids on bone mineral density and bone markers. More research is needed into the effects of inhaled corticosteroids, their impact on bone density and future fracture risk.

Osteoporosis appears to run in some families, but it seems that family history of fracture needs to be validated more widely before it can be included in a definitive list of risk factors. In women, exposure to oestrogen has been extensively studied; the age of menarche, any periods of amenorrhoea and the time of the menopause need to be taken into account. It also appears that oestrogen exposure has a different significance at different ages, which complicates a full understanding of this area. Hypogonadism in men is found as a secondary cause of osteoporosis, but as it is difficult to spot clinically it has limited value as a screening tool.

It is important that health professionals working in the areas where patients with the conditions and drug therapy associated with osteoporosis are seen are fully aware of these risks. Hyperparathyroidism and thyroid disease are associated with a reduced bone density. Immunosuppressant therapy and chronic anticonvulsant therapy (Compston and Rosen 1999) are associated with osteoporosis, and anyone who is exposed to these drugs must be considered at risk. Other conditions include malabsorption diseases, and the after-effects of organ transplantation.

Excess alcohol is a problem, especially in men, but this may be more to do with fracture risk. Smoking has not been found to be a risk factor in all epidemiological studies, but current smokers and those who have smoked heavily in the past appear to be at risk.

The effect of diet in osteoporosis is complicated, as a number of nutritional factors are thought to be important for bone health (Burns et al. 2003). Intake of calcium, vitamin D and protein should all be assessed. There is also growing evidence that fruits and vegetables are important for bone health (Burns et al. 2003). It is useful to assess dietary risk factors to enable the practitioner to give lifestyle advice; the healthy eating message for bone health is in line with international healthy eating advice. Physical activity is a modifiable risk factor for most individuals, but again there is conflicting evidence.

The interaction between the clinical risk factors and their usage and value in practice is difficult to evaluate. This can be partially understood by the prevalence of the various risk factors and their significance. For example, steroid use has a high predictive value for osteoporosis, but is rare in the population, which limits its value as a general screening tool. A low calcium intake or a low level of exercise, for example, are more commonly found in the population but are less predictive for osteoporosis. This means that the number of people who have a risk factor but will not be found to have osteoporosis is relatively high (false positives), and an unacceptable number of people without a risk factor will have osteoporosis (false negatives).

Does the number of risk factors a person has reflect an increased risk? There is some evidence that women who have five or more risk factors have an increased risk of fracture, but it is still contentious. Black et al. (2001) and Woolf and Akesson (2003) suggest that the exact interaction of risk factors is unclear.

Finding those patients at risk

As osteoporosis is generally a silent disease until fracture, and as general population screening is not currently recommended, a case-finding strategy could be used to find, assess and treat people at risk. One way to identify and treat people to prevent further fracture could be by using clinical risk factors to identify those at risk.

In primary care, options could include:

- using the read codes to identify those on steroids, those with previous fractures and those with certain conditions associated with osteoporosis
- using well women/men clinics to undertake screening of risk factors and provide health promotion advice
- including a question about falls in the last year in any encounter with older people.

In secondary care, health professionals involved with the conditions that are associated with osteoporosis need to be aware of the fact, counsel and, if appropriate, screen.

A fracture liaison service could be implemented. This involves setting in place a scheme to identify patients with low-trauma fractures. After a brief assessment, patients within set parameters (such as age range and type of fracture) are referred for a bone density scan. Following the scan they are seen and assessed by a specialist nurse who informs them of the results of the scan and gives health promotion advice. A letter is then sent to their GP, with advice on appropriate treatment and follow-up.

Rationale for consideration for bone densitometry

Although osteoporosis is such a common problem in people over 50, it is not felt that mass screening of the population is appropriate. This is because the current tests used to measure bone density will only identify half the people who have had fractures and are scanned as having a low bone density. There is no currently available method of assessing bone quality, a factor that we know probably contributes to 50% of bone fragility. This has led to the recommendation that assessment and treatment should be targeted at those at the highest risk; this is known as a case-finding strategy, as mentioned earlier.

The Royal College of Physicians (RCP 1999) suggests that people who have any of the following risk factors should be investigated for osteoporosis by having a dual X-ray absorptometry (DXA) scan:

- radiographic evidence of vertebral fracture
- radiographic osteopenia
- previous low-trauma limb fracture
- planned or current oral glucocorticoid therapy for 3 months or more at any dose
- presence of strong risk factors
- monitoring of therapy.

Diagnosing osteoporosis

The diagnosis of osteoporosis was agreed at a consensus meeting of the World Health Organization in 1994, in response to a request for such a diagnosis to be used for clinical trials of drugs used to treat osteoporosis. It was set at a T-score (see below) of –2.5 for postmenopausal women.

The T-score

As mentioned earlier, peak bone mass is achieved between the ages of around 25 and 40. In order to understand the normal distribution of peak bone mass, a large number of young adults were scanned. When these scans were plotted they formed a normal distribution curve, and this information forms the normal reference range. A T-score is a comparison of a person's bone density against the normal reference range and expressed as in terms of standard deviations from normal (see Fig. 2.5).

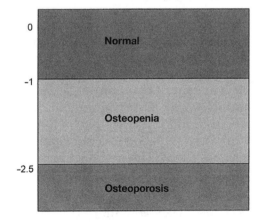

Figure 2.5 T-scores.

- Normal bone density is a T-score of above –1.
- Osteopenia (a low bone mass) has been defined as a T-score between –1 and –2. 5.
- Osteoporosis is a T-score below –2.5.

The Z-score

It is also possible to compare a person's bone density with an age-matched reference range, giving a Z-score, which is also expressed in standard deviations from the norm. Once a Z-score reaches –1 or lower there is an increase in fracture risk. The Z-score is used in children (who have not yet reached their peak bone mass) and elderly people, who would all fall into the osteoporosis category according to the T-score definition.

The concept of using an arbitrary threshold of bone density based on a comparison with young normal people to define osteoporosis does not do justice to the complexity of the disease. The classification of osteoporosis as a T-score of less than –2.5 is also used as an intervention threshold to start treatment, something for which it was not designed.

A better way of making treatment decisions could be a 10-year absolute fracture risk. Currently, work is being undertaken at an international level to produce this risk based on age, bone mineral density and other risk factors, and it is envisaged that in the near future risk tables similar to those produced for heart disease risk will be available.

Measuring bone density

Dual X-ray absorptometry (DXA)

Measurement can be made at both central and peripheral sites. Central DXA is the current 'gold standard' method and offers measurements taken at the sites of most serious fracture risk – the spine and the hips. The type of machine needed for central DXA (see Fig. 2.6) is not portable, so people have to travel to centres that have this equipment. Some machines are also able to use an instant vertebral assessment (IVA) function to assess vertebral fractures. This method of evaluating bone mineral density has a low radiation dose, good precision and accuracy, and the reference data have been validated. The machines are expensive, however, and the scans are dependent on good operator technique.

Peripheral DXA scanning

It is possible to measure the forearm or heel using a peripheral DXA

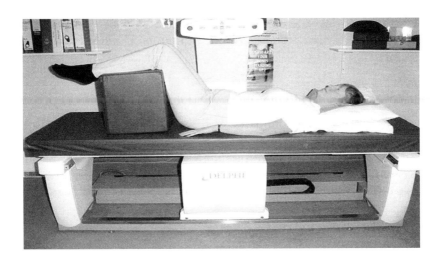

Figure 2.6 DXA scan.

machine, which is portable and less costly than a central DXA machine. The National Osteoporosis Society (2001) expert committee have evaluated the use of these machines and made recommendations that bone mineral density (BMD) of the heel (calcanus) is not routinely used, although it may have a place for screening. For DXA of the forearm, the following recommendations apply:

- If the T-score is less than –2.5 and the person has other risk factor/ previous fracture, then treatment may be indicated.
- If the T-score is between –1 and –2.5 then a central DXA scan of the lumbar spine and hips should be performed.
- If the T-score is above –1 and the person has not had a previous fracture, they should be reassured that their risk of future fracture is low.

Ultrasound

Ultrasound techniques, based on ultrasonic transmission through bone, are portable, quick and do not involve radiation. The technique consists of quantitative ultrasound (QUS) applied in the form of speed of sound (SOS) and broadband ultrasound attenuation (BUA). Ultrasound is not a measure of bone density in the way that DXA is, but rather a measure of other qualitative properties of bone, and may reflect the amount of bone present. The precision and stability may not be as good as DXA. Studies of QUS and association with osteoporotic fractures are mostly cross-sectional studies.

QUS cannot at present be used to diagnose osteoporosis as it is currently defined. Individuals who are found to have low QUS readings should be referred for a central DXA scan, or in the case of postmenopausal women may be advised to take preventive therapy if other major clinical risk factors are present.

Quantitative computed tomography (QCT)

This method offers true volumetric density measurements, but is limited by lower fracture predictability, higher radiation dose and higher cost. Also, the machine cannot scan the femur. The requirement for a calibration system, the cost of the scan and the increased radiation dose mean that at present this technique is not used in routine clinical practice.

Bone markers

These are biochemical markers of bone turnover, and can measure bone resorption and formation. During the bone remodelling process, breakdown products of collagen and enzymes are produced, travel into the circulation and are excreted in urine. Bone markers measure changes in resorption and include C- and N-telopeptides (CTX, NTX), and deoxypyridinoline (DPD) which can be detected in serum and urine. The markers of bone formation include osteocalcin and the procollagen type 1 propeptides C- and N-terminals, and also the enzyme bone alkaline phosphatase.

These biochemical markers are used to monitor response to treatment and are now becoming more widely available. They should not be used to diagnose osteoporosis. A sample of blood, or more commonly a second morning sample of urine, is taken to establish a person's baseline and then another sample collected in 3–6 months. The markers of bone resorption are usually suppressed by around 50% in the first 3 months of treatment. Undertaking this test can aid compliance, as the person can be told the drugs are having an effect, but currently it is not known how individual changes predict fracture risk.

There is also variability in measurements due to circadian variation, the seasons, menstrual cycle and food intake, which present differently in the markers. Work is currently ongoing to understand the variability.

Bone health promotion

It is well established that health is influenced by genetic, biological, lifestyle, environment and social factors. The Royal College of Physicians guidelines (RCP 1999) state that the modifiable risk factors such as lifestyle factors should be addressed in the prevention and management of osteoporosis.

An approach to healthy bones could work in the following areas: a universal approach to bone health, one targeted at those at high risk and one for those with osteoporosis.

Universal approach to bone health

Universal prevention is a whole-community approach, where everyone would eat a healthy diet throughout their life. This would require an adequate food supply, good nutrition policy and education. The health-related benefit of high consumption of fruit and vegetables has been established for a variety of body systems, including bone health.

The community would also need to understand the importance of bone health, and undertake an exercise programme that provides optimum bone health. An informed workforce of health professionals would be needed, and there would be a need to develop good communication for all age sectors of the population. There would also need to be an awareness of groups with an increased risk, and wide availability of education and nutritional advice. Local campaigns could be integrated into other initiatives, such as walking, diet, cookery clubs, and so on. Simple dietary guidelines for optimal bone health would have to be developed, e.g. three daily servings of calcium-rich foods for optimal bone health. There is also a need to combat the widespread perception that dairy foods should be avoid because they are fattening.

Although this does appear to be a rather utopian idea and in reality may not be likely to happen it, is certainly a goal that we should aim for if we are going to promote a positive approach to bone health.

High-risk groups

These groups would need to pay special attention to their diet and might need fortified foods or supplements. Preventive health services could include mobile ultrasound machines and screening targeted at risk populations. Prevention of fracture though accident in line with Standard Six of the National Service Framework for Older People and the recently published NICE guidelines (2004) would need to be addressed.

People with osteoporosis

Areas to be addressed would include:

- healthy eating advice, emphasizing the need to avoid the overconsumption of urinary calcium-wasting agents, such as salt and caffeine
- the role of exercise in helping to prevent fractures

- availability of help and information
- availability of safe and tolerable treatments with adequate information to make informed choices regarding treatment options.

Dietary factors and exercise

Addressing nutritional and dietary factors is complex. Biley (2002) reports that in older people the ability to achieve good nutrition is complicated by medication, ability to prepare food, self-esteem, the cost of food, and access to it (which includes the ability to travel to shops). Berg (2003) reports that nutritional change strategies have been found to be effective, if carried out in 2–3 individual or group sessions and at a medium intensity.

Calcium

Bone is the body's reservoir for calcium and it contains 99% of the body's calcium. The current recommendations are for a daily intake of 700 mg, in adults (see Table 2.2), but there is evidence that people with osteoporosis may need to boost their intake to 1200 mg. A number of sources also recommend that peri- and postmenopausal women should aim for 1000 mg a day. A poor calcium intake at any age can be a problem for the bones, but a very high calcium intake (above the recommended level) is not a guarantee against osteoporosis.

Table 2.2 Recommended daily calcium intake (mg)

Children (5–12 years)	500
Teenagers/young adults	800–1000
Adults (men and women)	700
Adults with osteoporosis	1200–1500 (including supplements if taken)

Based on the recommendations of the Department of Health Committee on Medical Aspects of Food and Nutrition Policy (COMA) 1998 (International Osteoporosis Society 2002). Reproduced by permission of HMSO.

A number of factors inhibit calcium; for example, a high intake of caffeine may affect calcium balance. When the diet is very high in protein, the protein is broken down to sulphuric acid and then neutralized by the body with calcium, sodium, potassium and other alkaline substances, which reduces the amount of these minerals for use in bone-building and may also increase the loss of calcium in the urine. Salt can also increase the amount of calcium excreted in the urine. It is not yet known how much salt intake can cause this problem, but intake should be limited to 6 g a day.

Vitamin D

Vitamin D is needed to absorb calcium into the bloodstream. The best source is sunlight. About 15–20 minutes in the sun with the arms and face uncovered, on every sunny day (being careful not to burn), will enable the body to make enough vitamin D for bone health. Vitamin D, which is fat soluble, is stored in the body. It is very difficult to eat enough vitamin D for bone health, although it is found in butter, margarine (where it is added as fortification) and oily fish. Vitamin D is also added to breakfast cereal and is found in cod liver oil.

Certain groups of people may be vulnerable to vitamin D deficiency. These include:

- Asian infants, young children and pregnant women on restricted diets
- Afro-Caribbean children on restricted diets
- people who stay indoors, especially residents of nursing and residential homes
- people who are always fully covered up by their clothing
- older people who eat no fish or meat (National Osteoporosis Society 2001).

Micronutrients

Eating a varied diet, including the recommended five portions of fruit and vegetables each day, will help to provide the micronutrients needed for bone health. Nuts and seeds also contain some micronutrients, such as copper and manganese.

Exercise

People who lead an active lifestyle have a higher bone density and a lower risk of fracture than those who are less active. Weight-bearing exercise increases bone density because of the force and load exerted on the bones during this exercise. Optimum bone health requires 30 minutes of weight-bearing exercise every day. The National Osteoporosis Society uses the concept of putting a jolt through the skeleton. They recommend brisk walking, jogging, scout's pace, skipping and jumping. (All the above activities should be performed safely, according to the usual advice given to people who are starting exercise.) Ambling around the shops for 30 minutes is not enough. For older people, or those with osteoporosis and/or fracture, the above advice would not be suitable. This group needs assessment and an exercise plan worked out with a properly qualified individual. Exercises may focus on the areas most likely to fracture – the wrist, spine and hip.

A number of sources support the importance of exercise. The Royal College of Physicians guidelines (RCP 1999) state that exercise increases well-being, muscle strength and postural stability and suggests exercise individually tailored to a selected group. Following a review of the evidence, Feder et al. (2000) state that individually tailored exercise programmes, delivered by qualified professionals to selected groups, do work. However, the best type and intensity of exercise, and the optimum time spent on it, is currently not known.

Investigations

Before starting people on treatment it is important to identify any causes of secondary osteoporosis that might need treatment. A clinician should also exclude other disease that may present as osteoporosis (e.g. malignancy or osteomalacia). Physical investigations may include:

- height
- kyphosis
- postural hypotension
- visual assessment
- cardiac
- neurological, body sway
- musculoskeletal
- feet (see Chapter 3 for further information).

The following tests may be undertaken:

- X-ray of lumbar/thoracic spine to rule out bony secondaries
- urea and electrolytes to exclude osteodystrophy
- calcium (to exclude osteomalacia or primary hyperparathyroidism)
- liver function to exclude alcohol abuse/chronic liver disease
- ESR
- thyroid function tests
- calcium, phosphate and alkaline phosphatase, which will be abnormal in osteomalacia, bony secondaries and hyperparathyroidism.

Depending on the context, further investigations may be undertaken to exclude conditions that mimic osteoporosis:

- electrophoresis, to rule out myeloma,
- testosterone, SHBG, undetected hypogonadism, PSA.

The role of physiotherapy in osteoporosis

Physiotherapy can be very useful for a person with osteoporosis. The physiotherapist can make a full assessment and offer back care advice. Advice can be given on specific exercises that target areas of high risk, and their work may include posture, balance and gait training. Work undertaken in New Zealand has shown that for someone with a very high risk of fracture individual tailored exercise, balance and gait training reduces both fall and fractures (Robertson et al. 2001). Hydrotherapy is a very good aid for those in pain, as it helps people to move joints and exercise muscle and can be offered by the physiotherapy department. Other methods of pain relief that may be available include transcutaneous electrical nerve stimulation (TENS) and acupuncture.

Drugs

The role of calcium and vitamin D

There is evidence that calcium supplementation at around 1 g/day slows the rate of bone loss in postmenopausal women, predominantly at sites of cancellous bone and mainly in the first year of intervention. A number of studies show a reduction in vertebral fracture rates in those given calcium supplements, and there is some evidence to suggest a reduction in hip fractures.

Calcium supplements are usually given with vitamin D. It appears from the evidence that in the poorly mobile, frail elderly population giving calcium and vitamin D supplements reduces fracture rates. In the UK, elderly and housebound people do not have enough vitamin D for bone health. As well as assisting in absorbing calcium from the intestinal tract, this vitamin is also needed for muscle and may well have a role in reducing falls. A low blood level of vitamin D may also lead to secondary hyperparathyroidism, leading to increased bone turnover and resorption of calcium from the bone.

Other drug treatments

The main group of drugs used to treat osteoporosis are bisphosphonates. These drugs inhibit the cells that break down the bone (osteoclasts) and allow the cells that rebuild bone (osteoblasts) to work more effectively. The second-generation bisphosphonates improve bone density and reduce vertebral fractures and non-vertebral fracture by around 50%. Bisphosphonates have poor bioavailability and bind to calcium. They should be taken on an empty stomach, with water. They also pose a risk of oesophageal irritation if they get stuck in the oesophagus, and it is recommended that they are washed down with a full glass of water and the person stays upright for 30 minutes to reduce this risk.

There are three oral bisphosphonates currently on the market in the UK:

- The second-generation agents alendronate and risedronate, available as either daily or weekly preparations. To reduce risks of gastro-oesophageal side effects, patients should be advised to swallow the tablet whole with a large glass of water when they get up in the morning, and remain fasting and stay upright for 30 minutes.
- The first-generation agent disodium etidronate (Didronel PMO) is available as a tablet to be taken for 2 weeks in a 3-month cycle and should be taken in the middle of a 4-hour fast, followed by a calcium supplement.

There has been little work comparing the bisphosphonates, but they work rapidly and show a fracture reduction within a year.

Intravenous bisphosphonates

Pamidronate is available as an infusion for those who cannot tolerate oral bisphosphonates or are not responding to them. It is given intravenously, and a reported side effect is acute phase reaction (flu-like symptoms).

Hormone replacement therapy (HRT)

Long-term use of HRT is no longer recommended for osteoporosis, although recent large studies have shown its effect on fracture reduction. It is currently recommended for use for early menopause or hysterectomy as bone protection, and can be given up to age of normal menopause. Because of the risk of side effects, a woman needs to be counselled on the risks and benefits of taking it. Once a woman stops taking HRT her bone density is back to where it would have been in 5 years had she not taken HRT.

Selective oestrogen receptor modulators (SERMs)

These were designed to mimic the action of oestrogen on certain receptors while blocking its effects on other receptors. A second-generation SERM, raloxifene (Evista), has been developed which provides protection against bone loss and reduces the incidence of vertebral fracture. It also reduces the risk of oestrogen-receptor breast cancer, does not stimulate the womb lining and appears to reduce some types of cholesterol, although there is no conclusive evidence of reductions in heart disease or stroke (research is continuing). There is a risk of deep-vein thrombosis, as with the contraceptive pill or HRT. The dosing regime is one 60-mg tablet tablet once a day, swallowed whole at any time.

Calcitonin

This is a hormone produced by the thyroid gland, which is involved in blood calcium balance. Some research studies have shown that it improves bone density, but there are no strong fracture data. It can be used to help reduce the pain following a vertebral fracture; it is given by subcutaneous injection or nasal spray.

Teriparatide (parathyroid hormone)

This hormone is naturally produced by the parathyroid gland. Intermittent low doses stimulate the osteoblasts to build more bone. It appears to work by encouraging the production of the osteoblasts whose work is then spread beyond the bone remodelling unit to increase the amount of bone built up. It is given as a daily subcutaneous injection, in a device similar to an insulin pen. Limitations include ability to inject, and cost.

Strontium ranulate (Protolos)

This is a new type of preparation, a dual action bone agent, which simultaneously increases bone formation and decreases bone resorption. It is licensed to reduce both vertebral and hip fractures. It comes as a 2-g sachet of granules which must be mixed with water before administration. Its gastrointestinal side effects are less than placebo, but it needs to be taken 2 hours after a calcium-containing foodstuff.

New areas of interest/drugs/formulations

The growth hormones are currently under investigation, with promising results in early studies particularly in young people with low bone mass including those with anorexia nervosa, demonstrating improvements in bone density and muscle mass and perhaps having a dual role in preventing fractures.

A new bisphosphonate, ibandronate, is likely to be available as a monthly tablet in the second half of 2005. This dosing regimen may benefit frail elderly people, as it would enable a health care worker to administer this drug correctly once a month.

Hip protectors

Hip protectors are pants into which is stitched a shell that covers the trochanteric region of the hip; hard-shell and soft-shell versions are available. In the case of a fall on the hip, the protector will shunt away the energy towards the soft tissues around the hip and the muscles around the femur.

The major limiting factor with hip protectors is compliance, because of their bulk and the need to wear them 24 hours a day. The pants need to be worn at night, as this is when a number of fractures occur. Other issues relating to poor compliance include poor fit, the extra effort required to wear the protectors, urinary incontinence and physical difficulties or illness. Compliance may be better with the soft-shell pants. Proper sizing and assessment of the patient is important.

Evidence suggests that hip protectors can reduce hip fractures in older people in institutional settings, but there is currently no evidence to support their use in community-dwelling populations (Parker et al. 2005). Given these factors, and despite poor long-term compliance, they are well worth trying in high-risk populations.

Guidance on the use of hip protectors

Guidelines have been provided in an effort to identify individuals who would benefit from hip protector pants. The guidelines below are used across the primary and secondary care interface in Southampton University Hospitals NHS trust and three local primary care trusts.

Who should be using hip protectors?

Following a review of the evidence, the District Falls Group recommend the use of hip protectors in:

- mobile people with a high risk of falling living in residential and nursing homes
- selected community-dwelling people at high risk of falling (not evidence based)

People who have had both hips replaced will not benefit from hip protectors. They should not be used for patients who have an active pressure sore over the hip area.

Assessing the patient

The use of hip protectors requires individual assessment of the patient including the following points:

- Compliance
- Continence assessment
- Correct measurement and fit
- Advice on use and laundering
- A 'trial run' to ensure the patient can take the pants up and down easily.

Good practice points

- Consider providing one pair of hip protectors with a follow-up within 1 week to assess compliance, etc. before the providing further garments.
- The patient should be encouraged to wear the hip protectors at night.
- The patient can wear ordinary pants under the hip protector pants; this may reduce the need for washing.
- If the patient has problems with incontinence, a shaped incontinence pad would need to be used.

Training

The provision of hip protectors needs to be supported by an education programme for staff involved with their issue and use. The planned implementation of 'falls champions' in residential and nursing homes provides an excellent opportunity for this (see Chapter 3).

Supply

Various types of hip protector are available. Types that require the shells to be removed for washing are not recommended. The Falls Group recommends the use of hip protectors that:

- are available in a wide range of styles and sizes
- can be washed at up to 35°C (95°F)
- are comfortable to wear for 24 hours.

Other guidelines and information

The National Institute for Clinical Effectiveness (NICE) is currently undertaking technology assessments in the area of osteoporosis. They are currently producing guidelines on secondary prevention (once a person has sustained a fracture). The aim of the guidelines is to inform the cost-effectiveness of treatments for osteoporosis to prevent fracture.

The National Osteoporosis Society is a charity that provides support to people with osteoporosis. They provide an excellent range of information booklets, a national telephone helpline and a network of local support groups. Their website can be found at *www.nos.org.uk*.

It is important that all health and social care professionals who are involved in the care and management of the patient with a hip fracture have a good awareness of secondary prevention in relation to osteoporosis. In meeting Standard Six of the National Service Framework for older people, it is also necessary to ensure that we aim to provide a model of delivery for a fully integrated falls and osteoporosis service. A recent publication by the All Party Parliamentary Osteoporosis Group (2004) has highlighted the blocks to the implementation of such services. This sets out the requirements of an osteoporosis service that can be slotted into an integrated falls and osteoporosis service. It is hoped that this will go some way towards clarifying service delivery models that will meet the requirements of Standard Six. In the following chapter consideration will be given to the prevention and management of falls, which are the major precipitating factor for hip fracture.

CHAPTER THREE

Falls in older people

A fall has been described as 'unintentionally coming to rest on the floor or some lower level, other than as a consequence of a violent blow, loss of consciousness or sudden onset of paralysis as in stroke or an epileptic seizure' (Kellogg International Group; Gibson et al. 1987). Many researchers have used this or similar definitions of a fall in their studies. However, other researchers have used a broader definition of falls to include those that occur as a result of dizziness or syncope (Lord et al. 2001). Defining falls in different ways can make comparisons between different studies difficult. It can also be of practical significance: for example, a trip or slip may not be reported as a fall, and someone who has inadvertently stumbled backwards onto a bed or chair may not consider themselves to have fallen (Perdue 2003). These issues need to be considered when attempting to understand the complex nature of falls in older people.

Falls are such a common problem in older people that they are considered to be one of the 'giants of geriatrics'. Each year in Britain a third of the population aged over 65 years has a fall, and half of those fall at least twice (Lord et al. 2001). Women are at greater risk of falling than men, with half of all women aged over 85 years in any one year having a fall (Blake et al. 1998). Falls are also the most common cause of death in adults over the age of 75 years, as well as being a significant cause of disability and injury (McMurdo et al. 2000, Smith 2000). Given these figures, it is therefore not surprising that the Department of Health has included falls prevention as Standard Six of the National Service Framework for Older People (DH 2001a). The aim of Standard Six is to reduce the prevalence of serious falls that cause injury, as well as to promote effective treatment and rehabilitation of those who have fallen.

The consequences of a fall may include fractures, most commonly in the humerus, pubic rami or hip, and admission to hospital. Even if people are uninjured as a result of a fall they may be unable to get up and could develop pressure sores, hypothermia or bronchopneumonia, or suffer dehydration. Psychological consequences include a fear of loss of independence and a fear of the reduction in quality of life (Salkeld et al. 2000, Murphy et al. 2003). Loss of confidence may also occur, with a resulting decrease in activity and increasing dependency. Falls are known to have a major impact on health and health care costs (Oliver et al. 2004) and are a major precipitating factor for admission to institutional care (Lord et al. 2001).

Risk factors for falls can be classified as intrinsic (e.g. visual deficits, balance disorders, functional and/or cognitive impairment), extrinsic (e.g. polypharmacy) and environmental. For the purpose of this chapter risk factors will be considered individually, but it is necessary to appreciate the complex interaction between multiple risk factors. The list of risk factors discussed in this chapter is not exhaustive, but helps to provide examples of the classifications highlighted above.

Environmental risk factors

The home, whether private or residential, is the most common place for falls to occur; 75% of deaths from falls occur in the home environment. Of these fatal falls, 60% occur on the stairs, resulting in almost 1000 deaths per year (Table 3.1, in DTI 1999). Examples of other hazards in the home include poor lighting, slick or irregular floor surfaces, trailing telephone cables, and furnishings or bathroom fixtures that are too high or too low. Studies examining environmental risk factors have generally demonstrated that modifying the home environment without altering other components of multifactorial interventions is not beneficial in reducing the risk of falls (Sattin et al. 1998, Cumming et al. 1999).

Extrinsic factors

The relationship between polypharmacy and falls is well established, but the relationship between specific classes of drugs and risk of falling is not so clear (Lord et al. 2001). An in-depth analysis of drug classes and falls in older people is beyond the scope of this chapter, but it is important to recognize that certain drug groups have been most commonly implicated in the aetiology of falls.

Several groups of medicines have been associated with the risk of hip fracture, and some of these also contribute to falls in older people. Furosemide, because of its action of promoting calcium excretion by the kidneys, may expose users to an increased risk of osteoporosis and osteoporotic fractures (Tromp et al. 2000). Furosemide and thiazide diuretics can also increase the risk for syncope, but thiazide diuretics may have a positive effect on bone density, by decreasing excretion of calcium in the kidney, which could reduce the risk of hip fracture (Jones et al. 1995).

Table 3.1 Total number of fatal falls in the home in the UK: 1995–1997

	Under 65			Over 65		Total
	0–14	15–39	40–64	65–74	75+	
Men						
Between two levels	5	7	20	15	55	102
From building	8	40	31	16	29	124
From ladder	0	2	39	49	38	128
On same level	0	3	14	16	53	86
On stairs or steps	3	66	267	182	321	839
Unspecified	5	29	224	196	735	1189
	21	147	595	474	1231	2468
Total men						
%	0.9	6	24	19	50	
%		31			69	100
Women						
Between two levels	2	1	9	22	153	187
From building	4	12	7	8	18	49
From ladder	0	0	6	4	5	15
On same level	0	1	14	26	121	162
On stairs or steps	3	44	161	134	402	744
Unspecified	1	10	127	214	1797	2149
	10	68	324	408	2496	3306
Total women						
%	0.3	2	10	12	75	
%		12			88	100
All						
Between two levels	7	8	29	37	208	289
From building	12	52	38	24	47	173
From ladder	0	2	45	53	43	143
On same level	0	4	28	42	174	248
On stairs or steps	6	110	428	316	723	1583
Unspecified	6	39	351	410	2532	3338
	31	215	919	882	3727	5774
Total all						
%	0.5	4	16	15	65	
%		20			80	100

Note : Because of rounding percentages may not add up to 100
Source : Metra Martech

Source: DTI (1999) Avoiding Slips, Trips and Broken Hips. Reproduced with kind permission of HMSO.

In all settings (e.g. community, long-term care, hospital and rehabilitation) there is a consistent association between the use of psychotrophic medications (i.e. neuroleptics, benzodiazepines and antidepressants) and falls. The relative risk of hip fracture among long-term users of long elimination half-life benzodiazepines was 1.7 compared to the risk of 1.1 for those using benzodiazepines with a short half-life, irrespective of differences in age, gender, nursing home residence, previous hospital admissions, use of other antihypertensive drugs, body mass, ambulatory status, functional status or dementia (Cumming and Klineber 1993).

Medications associated with postural hypotension that may contribute to the risk of falls include diuretics, antihypertensives, antiparkinsonian and antianginal agents. The sedative effects of agents such as hypnotics, antihistamines and opioid analgesics may also contribute to the risk of falls in older people. Other side effects that may occur as a result of taking medications such as amlodipine and nonsteroidal anti-inflammatory drugs (NSAIDs) include dizziness, and imbalance may occur as a result of taking phenothiazines and prochlorperazine. Physiological mechanisms underlying the association between medications and falls are complex and include changes in the central nervous system, postural hypotension, lack of neuromuscular coordination and impaired balance.

The complex interaction of medications taken by older people and their potential side effects should therefore be carefully considered when attempting to reduce the risk of falls. Medications should be regularly reviewed, with the type and number of medications being identified. Unnecessary medication should be stopped and inappropriate doses adjusted. Care must be taken to balance the benefits and risks associated with the withdrawal of certain medications; for example, discontinuing antihypertensive drugs to prevent the risk of falls is not warranted in most cases because the risk of morbidity due to hypertension is high and evidence between the use of antihypertensive drugs and falls is weak (Stegman 1983, cited in Lord et al. 2001). Careful prescribing should be advocated, with avoidable risk factors being taken into consideration. Involving the patient, carers and family members is obviously essential and should include a discussion of whether and how drugs are being taken.

There appear to be no randomized controlled studies of manipulation of medication as a sole intervention for the reduction of falls risk. In multifactorial studies, reduction of medications was found to be a prominent component of effective falls-reducing interventions in community-based and long-term care facilities. These studies suggest that a reduction in the number of medications in patients who are taking more than four preparations is beneficial (Campbell et al. 1999, Close et al. 1999).

Intrinsic factors

Visual impairment

Visual impairment is strongly associated with risk of falling and hip fracture (Ivers et al. 1998, Abdelhafiz and Austin 2003). This association may be explained by poor visual acuity, reduced visual field, impaired contrast sensitivity and cataract (Ivers et al. 1998). Visual impairment is defined as a level of vision below the level an individual requires for everyday tasks. A common cut-off point is taken as binocular visual acuity of 6/12 or 6/18 (Evans et al. 2002).

Causes of visual impairment include refractive errors, cataracts, diabetes, glaucoma, macular degeneration and visual field loss. It has been suggested that with the application of current knowledge significant reduction of visual impairment may be attained when the impairment is caused by refractive errors, diabetes mellitus, cataract or glaucoma (Van Newkirk et al. 2001). In the case of macular degeneration, treatment options are limited.

Evidence suggests that some older people are reluctant to attend for routine eye examinations, either for financial reasons, or because of a fear of being told bad news or because they believe poor eyesight is an inevitable consequence of ageing (Smeeth and Illiffe 1998). Health inequalities exist, with older people from lower socioeconomic groups being less likely to make use of community ophthalmic services (Jones et al. 1996). Potential eye problems may also be overlooked in older people in nursing homes and residential care, although they are known to be at increased risk of falls (van der Pols et al. 2000, Abdelhafiz and Austin 2003).

Recommendations made by the College of Optometrists and the British Geriatric Society, with endorsement by the Royal College of General Practitioners (COP/BGS 2003), include the need to ensure that screening for visual impairment becomes an integral part of a falls assessment, with those identified as suffering visual impairment having a full eye examination by an optometrist. Mechanisms to achieve this would need to be agreed locally and could take place in a variety of settings, with the needs of older people in residential care and nursing homes also being recognized and included in local service arrangements. It is also important to optimize the visual environment, remove physical hazards, and reduce other falls risk factors for older people with impaired vision.

Podiatry and foot care

The role of podiatry and the importance of foot care have often been given less consideration than other risk factors, although foot pain, biomechanical deformities, balance and gait problems are known to predispose people to an increased risk of falling. Inappropriate footwear may compound some of these problems, and with an estimated 80% of older people having one or more foot problems (Harvey et al. 1997, Helford et al. 1998) it is important that these factors are taken into consideration when falls risk assessments are undertaken. Significantly, Standard Six of the National Service Framework for Older People includes the need for podiatry to be included when NHS trusts set up specialist falls services.

Foot pain and the risk of falls are clearly linked, primarily because foot pain will cause a person to walk more slowly and experience greater difficulty in carrying out activities of daily living. Moreover, older people with foot pain are less able to balance and maintain coordination, especially when attempting to negotiate stairs. This is particularly relevant when considering the number of fatalities that occur as a result of falls on stairs. Proprioception can also become impaired as a result of plantar hyperkeratosis, and this may also contribute to the risk of falling (Menz and Lord 2001).

Deformities such as hammer toes and hallux valgus can be corrected surgically, and this will dramatically improve function of the older foot. This type of procedure can often be performed as day case surgery, and providing there is an adequate vascular supply to the foot this is suitable for many older people. Accurate diagnosis and interventions can help to maximize the function of the older foot.

Much of the advice for good foot care does not require specialist podiatric knowledge. For example, tips for foot health can be provided by any member of the multi-professional team working in acute and primary care settings. In the author's own area, primary and acute care staff have worked with the podiatry service to develop our 'top tips for foot health' (Box 3.1) which can be used with older people who do not have special foot care needs, for example diabetics.

Box 3.1 10 top tips for foot health

1 Wash feet daily, and dry well between the toes.
2 Don't soak feet for more than 10 minutes: it can make them dry.
3 Don't use talc between your toes: it clogs the pores.
4 File hard skin and corns – never use sharp objects to remove hard skin.
5 Use corn plasters with caution – they contain acids which can damage healthy skin.
6 Change footwear regularly and hosiery daily: this helps prevent athlete's foot and 'smelly feet'.
7 Your nails will be softer and easier to cut after you have had a bath.
8 Always cut nails straight across, and don't cut them lower than the end of the toe.

9 Never cut down the sides of the nail: this can cause painful ingrowing toenails.

10 Afterwards, clean your instruments in warm soapy water and dry them thoroughly.

Practical footwear advice (Box 3.2) can assist an older person to maintain stability, mobility and safety.

Box 3.2 Footwear advice

- Footwear should be selected for comfort and fit. This is essential to maintain your stability, mobility and safety.
- As we get older our feet change shape and size. It is important that you have your feet measured every time you buy shoes.
- Avoid high heels.
- Wear properly fitting, sturdy shoes that provide support.
- Shoes that fasten with laces or buckles are safer than slip-ons, but make sure the laces are tied. If you cannot tie laces, try shoes with a Velcro fastening instead.
- The sole of your shoe should be non-skid. Textured or rubber soles are usually best. Do not wear extra-thick soles, which can make you clumsy and increase your risk of falling.
- Wear slippers with non-slip soles. Slippers with Velcro or zip fastenings are best.
- Change slippers that are loose or out of shape.
- Never walk about with nothing or just stockings/socks on your feet.
- If you have difficulty obtaining a well-fitting pair of shoes, or can't get to the shops to buy shoes, there are some very good mail order footwear companies.

Simple measures in relation to footwear can achieve positive results. For example, one primary care trust pioneered a scheme whereby they negotiated a discount on slippers with fastenings and strong soles that provide enough support to reduce the risk of tripping and slipping and distributed about 100 pairs of these to residents in two nursing homes. Mulholland (2003) reports that the scheme to 'bin sloppy slippers' helped to reduce falls among older people by 60%. Footwear risk assessments can be used to guide and assist professionals with clinical judgements, and also in deciding the appropriateness of referral for specialist podiatry input. Studies relating to footwear examining falls as an outcome are limited. However, some trials have reported improvements in intermediate outcomes, such as balance, from specific footwear interventions. Results of timed mobility tests and functional reach were better when women wore walking shoes instead of being barefoot (Arnadottir and Mercer 2000). Static and dynamic balance were better in low-heeled rather than in high-heeled shoes or the individual's own footwear (Lord and Bashford 1996). Studies in men have shown that foot position awareness and stability are better with high mid-sole hardness and low mid-sole thickness (Robbins et al. 1997).

Exercise and balance

Exercise and balance programmes have been associated with improvements in falls prevention (Campbell et al. 1997, AGS/BGS/AAOP 2001) However, the best type, duration and intensity of exercise for falls prevention remain unclear, particularly when the heterogeneity of older people at risk of falling and the multifactorial nature of falls are taken into consideration. In a community population of relatively fit older people, a programme of very intensive strength and endurance exercises reduced the risk of subsequent falls and the proportion of fallers (Buchner et al. 1997). A randomized control trial demonstrated that in older community-dwelling women, individually designed exercise programmes in the home that incorporated strength and balance training reduced both falls and injuries (Campbell et al. 1999). A community-based generic exercise programme in older men was of no benefit in falls reduction (Rubenstein et al. 2000) and an individually designed exercise programme for nursing home residents with moderate dementia did not reduce falls (Mulron et al. 1994).

Cardiovascular disease

Some falls are considered to have a cardiovascular origin that may be amenable to intervention strategies often directed to syncope; for example, medication review and change or cardiac pacing. There can be an overlapping of symptoms of falls and syncope and a causal association between some cardiovascular disorders and falls, particularly orthostatic hypotension, carotid sinus syndrome and vasovagal syndrome (Dey et al. 1997, Richardson et al. 1997). In particular, up to 30% of older people with carotid sinus syndrome present with falls and have amnesia for loss of consciousness when bradyarrhythmia is induced experimentally (Kenny et al. 2001, Kumar et al. 2003).

Neurological problems

Several neurological problems, including stroke disease, which is common in older people, contribute to their risk of falling. In the case of a stroke disease, many people have difficulty in coordinating the actions of different muscle groups and cannot generate enough force in lower limb muscle groups (Moseley et al. 1993, cited in Lord et al. 2001). This may result in difficulty in maintaining leg extension on standing, and reduced foot clearance that may result in tipping. Gait difficulties following a stroke can also make it difficult for people to adapt to negotiating uneven ground and obstacles. Other parts of the brain that have been damaged as a result of a stroke can produce difficulties with balance, sensory and visual inattention, and can affect judgement. All of these factors can, in different ways, contribute to the risk of falls.

Other neurological conditions that increase the risk of falling are Parkinson's disease, peripheral neuropathy, myelopathy, cerebellar disorders and vestibular pathology (Lord et al. 2001).

Urinary incontinence

As will become apparent in Chapter 5, urinary incontinence is a common problem in older people, particularly in older women. Various studies have demonstrated the relationship between urinary incontinence and risk of falling (Luukinen et al. 1996, Stevenson et al. 1998). Most falls are thought to occur as a result of loss of balance when rushing to the toilet, or because of slipping on urine. However, it has been suggested that urinary incontinence may not be the primary cause of a fall but should be considered as more of a generalized marker of physical frailty, with the close association between incontinence, depression, falls and level of mobility suggesting that these interrelated symptoms may have shared risk factors rather than causal connections (Tinnetti et al. 1995).

Dementia

Recent studies continue to demonstrate the association between dementia and risk of falling (Cameron et al. 2002, Van Doorn et al. 2003). The environment, cardiovascular problems, medication and disturbances of balance and gait are factors that contribute to the significant risk of falling in this patient group. Treatment of these risk factors can reduce the risk of falls in cognitively normal older people (Shaw and Kenny 1998).

Given that people with dementia are more likely to fall than other older people, it is important to consider various prevention strategies and the contribution that they can make to reduce the risk of falling in this particularly vulnerable group. Currently there appears to be a paucity of research in this area, perhaps partly due to a reluctance to undertake research involving demented patients because of ethical considerations. However, research undertaken at the University of Newcastle, aimed at determining the effectiveness of multifactorial intervention after a fall in patients with cognitive impairment and dementia attending an accident and emergency department, concluded that preventive strategies were not effective in reducing the number of falls in people with dementia (Shaw et al. 2003). It could therefore be argued that the scarce resources available to implement falls prevention strategies should be channelled into tackling risk factors among older people who do not have dementia. However, as the population ages, the contribution from patients with dementia to the institutional and hospitalization costs as a result of a fall will continue to rise. The challenge of preventing falls in those with dementia will be ever present, and it is therefore essential that research in this area is encouraged and given high priority.

Preventing a 'long lie'

As previously suggested, some older people who fall will not sustain an injury but can be affected in other ways. One consequence of a fall is a 'long lie', which has been described as a period of one hour or more lying on the floor after a fall (Lord et al. 2001). During this period of time a person is susceptible to the development of pressure sores, hypothermia and pneumonia. They may also be in pain, miss medications or meals, become dehydrated and fatigued, be incontinent, suffer joint stiffness and become increasingly frightened and anxious.

Guidelines for the collaborative, rehabilitative management of fallers, put together by physiotherapists and occupational therapists, include preventing the consequence of a long lie. This can be achieved by teaching people how to get up from the floor, teaching them how to get help and teaching them coping strategies (for example, how to keep warm, change position and use a cushion to urinate into). For people who cannot get up from the floor without help, the use of a personal alarm which allows them to notify a person nearby or contact an operator who can arrange for appropriate assistance to be provided can be helpful in preventing long lies. Other actions included in guidelines are improving the safety of the surroundings, improving older people's ability to withstand threats to their balance and optimizing their confidence in their ability to move about safely and independently (CSP/COT 2000).

Research and cooperation

The complexity and dynamic interaction between intrinsic, extrinsic and environmental risk factors associated with falls in older people should not be underestimated. As highlighted in a recent Cochrane review, interventions to prevent falls that are likely to be effective are available, although there is a suggestion that less is known about their effectiveness in preventing falls-related injuries. Other areas of unknown effectiveness, such as those using a cognitive–behavioural approach, require further research (Gillespie et al. 2004).

Research undertaken by Help the Aged into the development of falls prevention service measured against the milestones of the National Service Framework for Older People has highlighted the varying stages of progress in different parts of the country, with some evidence of cross-agency partnership resulting in a well-integrated falls service. Meeting the government's milestones is dependent on the local priority of falls prevention (Help the Aged 2003). However, budget holders in health and social care agencies should be striving towards making falls prevention and rehabilitation an urgent priority, not only because of National Service Framework milestones that need to be met, but because of the impact that falls have on older people living in our society and those who care for them.

Falls in the hospital environment

Given the multifactorial risks associated with falls in older people, it is perhaps not surprising that falls remain a key issue in hospital settings. Evidence relating to the number of falls that occur in hospitals is limited, although it has been suggested that approximately 2% of older patients fall during their hospital stay (Mahoney 1998) and approximately 30% of such falls result in an injury (Oliver 2004).

Risk factors associated with falls in hospital are largely similar to those in the community. However, it is important to recognize that other significant factors come into play in an acute care environment. For some patients the risk of falling will remain throughout their stay, but for others the risk may be significantly increased at certain points during hospitalization; for example, if they develop an acute delirium postoperatively. A patient may be exposed to an increased risk of falling when independence is promoted as part of their rehabilitation programme (Perdue 2003).

A study by Frels et al. (2002) demonstrated significant risk predictors of falling as a history of a previous fall, benzodiazepine intake and the need for maximum assistance. Salgado et al. (1994) were able to correctly classify 80% of patients into faller and non-faller groups using four key variables: impaired orientation, psychoactive drug use, evidence of stroke and impaired performance on 'get up and go' test (standing up from a chair, walking 5 metres, turning around and returning to the chair). In a case control study of 232 hospital patients (Oliver et al. 1997), different but related predictors of falls were identified as a history of previous falls, reduced mobility and transfer skills, agitation and the need for frequent toileting.

Identifying those at risk of falling is a key component of any integrated approach to the prevention and management of falls in hospital. Other components include modification of risk factors, environmental risk factors, increasing awareness of falls risk and the reduction of injury from falls (Lord et al. 2001). The remainder of this chapter will focus on the development in the author's trust of an integrated approach to the identification, prevention and management of falls in hospital, in relation to the components identified by Lord and his colleagues.

Falls Group strategy

A Falls Group has been established in this acute trust since 2001, with representatives from directorates throughout the trust. There is also multi-professional representation from medicine, nursing and allied health professionals, and the group is chaired by a member of the clinical risk department. Meetings are held monthly and the aim of the Falls Group is to act as a forum in which to explore different perspectives on the management of falls, leading towards a consensus and more holistic approach to the care of patients, addressing recommendations from the National Service Framework for Older People and other relevant government guidelines (Box 3.3).

Box 3.3 Trust Falls Group philosophy statement

Falls management requires a multi-professional, trust-wide approach to ensure that all reasonable measures are taken to minimize the risk and number of falls, through a coordinated approach by:

- Risk assessment of all patients considered at risk of falls to identify those at high risk due to age or poor health
- Falls management reflected in a care plan/pathway
- Completion of adverse event form and pro-forma when a fall occurs and analysis of trending and learning lessons
- Education and training programme for patients, carers and staff.

As in many other hospital trusts, falls are a common occurrence in our hospital wards. Within the hospital trust, falls sit as the most reported incident, providing a significant percentage of the overall number of reported clinical incidents per month. A key objective of the Falls Group is to ensure that all staff are aware of the need to carry out an initial and updated falls risk assessment on patients at risk of falls, using a validated tool. We use STRATIFY (the St Thomas Risk Assessment Tool in falling elderly inpatients). This was selected because in two large cohort studies of 1217 and 331 patients it showed high sensitivity (correctly identified people as fallers) and good specificity (correctly identified people as non-fallers). Any risk assessment tool may be less effective in settings or patient populations different from those used in the index study, and this appears to be the case with STRATIFY, with the score being progressively less effective in settings remote from the original validation cohort (Oliver et al. 2004). However, because there are so few risk assessment tools with widespread validation we continue to use STRATIFY (Box 3.4), despite some difficulties particularly in relation to the calculation of the transfer and mobility score. Staff in several units throughout the trust have experienced these difficulties, and as a result a key objective for 2005 is to pilot and validate a new risk assessment tool which has been developed by our own Falls Group.

Box 3.4 STRATIFY fall risk assessment tool

1 Did the patient present to hospital with a fall, or has he or she fallen on the ward since admission?
(Yes = 1, No = 0)

Do you think the patient is (questions 2–5):
2 Agitated?
(Yes =1, No = 0)

3 Visually impaired to the extent that everyday functioning is affected?
(Yes = 1, No = 0)

4 In need of especially frequent toileting?
(Yes = 1, No = 0)

5 Transfer or mobility score of 3 or 4?
(Yes = 1, No = 0)

Total score:

Source: BMJ (1997); 315: 1049–53. Reproduced with kind permission from the BMJ Publishing Group.

A core care plan (Fig. 3.1) has been developed for patients who are identified as being at high risk of falls – this can be adapted to meet specific needs of individual patients. When falls occur in the ward environment, as well as completing an adverse event form, staff are also expected to complete a falls incident pro-forma (Fig. 3.2) in order to enable the clinical risk department to evaluate incidence of falls and causal factors.

Patient Addressograph		Ward: _____
Name		Care plan for maintaining safety (including risk of falling)
Hospital No.		
	Date: _____	Nurse signature: _____

Problem	Goal	Action	Review Date
.... is unable to maintain their own safety due to .... and has been assessed at risk of falling following STRATIFY risk assessment.	If bed bound – to maintain patient safety and reduce the risk of falling out of bed. If mobile – to maintain patient safety and reduce the risk of falls when mobilizing around the ward and unit area.	1. Encourage independence within limits of current ability. 2. Discuss with .... how they are at risk of injury and falling. 3. Encourage patient and family to discuss with nursing staff their concerns. 4. Encourage patient to co-operate with nursing staff and accept assistance when required. 5. Complete manual handling assessment. Use patient's own aids. (add details) .... 6. Refer to physiotherapist. 7. Nurse in observation bed. 8. Ensure the nurse call bell is within easy reach and the patient can use it. If unable, provide another means for patient to summon help. 9. Only use cot sides following risk assessment as per Trust policy. Cot sides in use: Yes/No 10. If patient tries to get out of bed unaided then consider nursing them on the floor. Discuss with multidisciplinary team, complete a risk assessment and then seek family's understanding. 11. Use pillows to support the patient and pad hard surfaces, unless contraindicated, e.g. spinal injury 12. Ensure patient wears slippers/shoes when out of bed. 13. Ensure bed space is free from hazards and adequately lit. 14. Escort the patient when mobilising; ensure patient understands the need to wait for staff to assist. 15. Orientate to day, time and place at all times. 16. Consider use of hip protectors. 17. Complete any adverse event forms. Keep family informed of accidents.	

Figure 3.1 Core care plan.

FALLS INCIDENT PRO-FORMA

NB: This form should be completed at the same time as the adverse event form (AEF) and <u>sent attached to it</u> to the Risk Management department as normal.

PATIENT ADDRESSOGRAPH	Ward:
	Date of admission:
	Date of fall:
	Time of fall:
	A.E.F. Report No:

<u>1. Details of Patient Fall</u>
   a) **Contributory Factors:**

   Wet floor ☐   Lack of staff ☐ Staff Sickness   ☐ Busy take   ☐

   Crisis on ward (arrest)   ☐ Ward round in progress ☐

   Other, please state...............................

   b) **Observed:**   Witnessed ☐   Not witnessed   ☐

2. <u>Controls in Place</u>:
   a) **COTSIDES IN PLACE (in position of use):**   Yes ☐   No ☐
   b) **RISK ASSESSMENT CARRIED OUT?**   Yes ☐   No ☐

Figure 3.2 Falls Incident pro-forma.

3. Impact upon Patient

    a) **TREATMENT REQUIRED:**   Xray ☐   Dressing ☐   POP ☐

    Surgery ☐   Referral to other specialist ☐

    b) **EXTENSION LENGTH OF STAY**   Days ☐   Weeks ☐   Months ☐

    (Likely/ anticipated)   Loss of nursing/rest home placement ☐

4. Patient Status at time of incident

    a) **PATIENT'S VIEW:**

    Needed to void ☐   Could not access nurse call ☐   Boredom ☐

    Confusion ☐   Walking aid not accessible ☐   Nurses too busy ☐

    b) **PATIENT'S MENTAL STATE:**

    Alert/orientated ☐   Acute confusional state ☐   Chronic confusional state ☐

    Dementia ☐

Figure 3.2 Falls Incident pro-forma (continued).

This documentation is used in all adult wards throughout the trust, and there is an accompanying poster on each of the wards which provides a clear pathway to be followed in the management of elderly people who fall. The poster also provides information on defining postural hypotension, postural blood pressure monitoring and referral to community falls services. The information is also printed on the back of each care plan (Fig. 3.3). A named 'falls champion' for each directorate has been identified and their name and bleep number is identified on the poster. A falls discharge checklist has also been developed for use in the emergency department (Fig. 3.4).

Risk factor modification

Having identified patients who are at increased risk of falling, it is important to attempt to modify risk factors that contribute to falls in the ward or clinical environment. A patient who presents with a fall should have a careful assessment of the reason for the fall, and may need to undergo thorough medical screening as the fall may be a symptom of an underlying pathology that can be treated. As previously suggested, review of medication is extremely important, and in our trust all older people admitted to an acute ward have their medication reviewed by the ward pharmacist in conjunction with medical staff. Other risk factors such as confusion, agitation, co-morbidity, reduced muscle strength, poor balance and poor vision should be investigated and addressed. Physiotherapy interventions and occupational therapy involvement may also be required, particularly when considering discharge home.

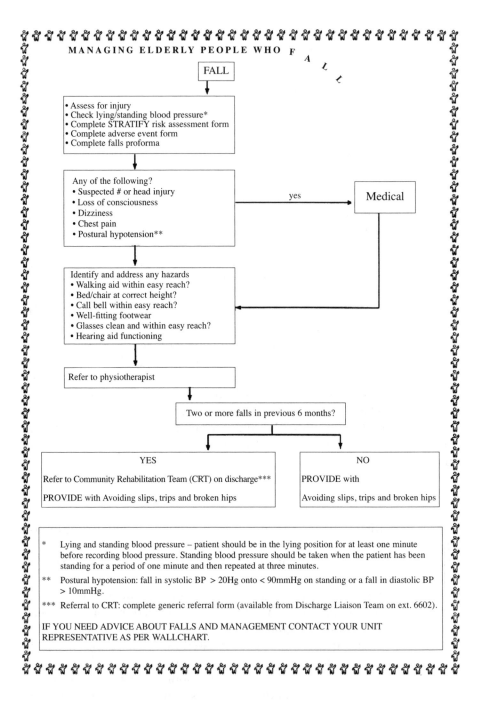

Figure 3.3 Managing elderly people who fall.

PATIENT ADDRESSOGRAPH	Date:
	Time:
	Name of Dr./nurse attending:

1. First fall: Y/N

If 'no', number of falls in previous year   ☐   * see
below

2. Fall associated with loss of consciousness/dizziness: Y/N

If 'yes', refer to Syncope Service (consultation card PLUS EGG)   ☐

If 'yes', refer to DVLA handbook for appropriate advice about driving   ☐

3. Could the patient get up after the fall (with/without help)   Y/N

If 'no', provide patient with information on how to summon help   ☐

4. Is the patient on any of the following drugs (tick boxes):

- sedatives (diazepam, temazepam)   ☐
- antipsychotics (haloperidol, risperidone)   ☐
- drugs for Parkinson's disease   ☐
  (Madopar, Sinemet, ropinirole, cabergoline)
- tricyclic antidepressants (amitriptyline)   ☐
- anticholinergic drugs (oxybutinin, tolterodine)   ☐
- cardiovascular drugs   ☐
  (diuretics, β-blockers, calcium blockers, ACE inhibitors)

If on 4 or more of the above, MEDICATION REVIEW BY THE GP IS ADVISED

5. Blood pressure: lying   standing/sitting:

(Postural hypotension on standing, drop in systolic blood pressure of ≥ 20 mmHg or any drop in systolic blood pressure below 90 mmHg or drop in diastolic blood pressure ≥ 10 mmHg

Postural hypotension   Y/N

If 'yes', provide patient with advice leaflet for postural hypotension.   ☐
MEDICATION REVIEW BY GP ADVISED

6. Fracture: Y/N

If 'yes', GP TO ASSESS OSTEOPOROSIS RISK

7. Difficulty recognising an object across a room or with reading   Y/N

If 'yes', advise patient to visit their optician   ☐

Figure 3.4 Falls discharge checklist.

8. Get Up & Go Test: Normal/abnormal

If 'abnormal', physiotherapist to assess gait prior to discharge

9. Evidence of poor footcare   Y/N

If 'yes', refer to podiatrist

10. Badly-fitting footwear   Y/N

If 'yes', advise patient to change footwear (Cosyfeet leaflet)

**PROVIDE THE PATIENT WITH HEALTH PROMOTION & FALLS ADVICE
LEAFLETS.**

PLEASE FAX THIS FORM TO THE PATIENT'S GP NOW.

***IF THE NUMBER IN THIS BOX IS > 1 PLEASE FAX THIS FORM
TO THE COMMUNITY DISCHARGE LIAISON TEAM (8684) NOW.**

SIGNATURE: _____

Figure 3.4 Falls discharge checklist (continued).

Environmental interventions

The hospital ward can present many hazards for the patient who is at risk of falling, and all staff must take every reasonable step to reduce the risk of falling and the consequence of falls. Falls awareness and prevention should be an integral part of maintaining a safe environment for patients. Floor spaces should be kept free from clutter and trailing cables. Spillages should be dealt with promptly, and warning signs that can be a potential hazard should be removed quickly. Equipment such as brakes on beds, commodes and wheelchairs should be regularly inspected and maintained. All staff can take simple precautions to reduce the risk of falls: for example, the nurse call bell should be within easy reach of the patient, as should other things that they might need such as a drinking glass and water. A patient stretching to reach for a glass that is not close at hand can easily fall from the bed. Beds and chairs should be at the correct height for transfer (these can be measured by occupational therapists). A simple but effective system is then to colour-code chairs according to their height, so that chairs of the correct height are given to patients according to their identified need. When patients are mobilizing it is important to ensure that they have their own mobility aid within easy reach. Although it can be argued that the mobility aid may contribute to the clutter around the patient's bed, which in itself is a risk factor, attempting to mobilize without the correct mobility aid poses a far greater risk of falling. Strategies employed to prevent people from falling should not prevent them from mobilizing if they are able to do so. The unnecessary restriction on standing and movement can contribute to greater losses of balance, strength and function which can in turn increase the potential for falling (Lord et al. 2001).

The use of side rails for those considered at risk of falling has proved controversial, with evidence highlighting the risks of using side rails particularly for acutely confused patients (Gray and Gaskell 1990, Everett and Bridel-Nixon 1997). Potential problems include the risk of entrapment and of falling from a greater height if the patient attempts to climb over the side rails. There are, however, circumstance when side rails can be of benefit: for example, when a cognitively intact person uses them as a mobility aid in bed. In our own trust a policy on side rails has been implemented, and this has assisted staff in undertaking a risk assessment when the use of side rails is under consideration. Obviously it is not only nursing staff who deal with patients, and on the trauma and elderly-care units a simple but effective way of dealing with this situation is to have a sign over each patient's bed highlighting that a risk assessment had been undertaken and whether or not side rails were to be used. As part of the risk assessment includes discussion with the patient, family and carers, consent is always obtained before displaying this sign. The use of these signs has now been adopted throughout the trust.

Increasing awareness of falls risk

To raise falls awareness throughout the trust, careful consideration had to be given to the education of all staff. A falls education training pack has been developed. The session takes approximately one hour to deliver, using a PowerPoint presentation or overhead projector, and the training pack is regularly updated to take national and local practice guidelines into account. A Falls Awareness Week is held once a year throughout the trust, and identified 'falls champions' in each directorate take responsibility for delivering falls education in their own area. This not only involves ward-based staff but also embraces areas such as portering and pharmacy services.

Reducing falls injury

Even with falls prevention in place, it is important to recognize that falls will still occur in the ward environment and appropriate measures should be taken to minimize the severity of falls-related injury. As highlighted in the previous chapter, hip protectors are increasingly being used to reduce fractured neck of femur, which is one serious consequence of falling. Although there is evidence to support the use of hip protectors in older people who require long-term care (Parker et al. 2005), no study investigating the use of hip protectors in community dwellers or acute care environments has yet been published. It is therefore difficult to recommend their wholesale use in the prevention of hip fractures in acute wards. The cost (about £40 per pair) may also be prohibitive. Shock-absorbing floor surfaces, sensor alarms which are activated when a potential faller is attempting to move, low beds and mattresses on the floor can also be used in the attempt to reduce injury from a fall.

Audit

For any falls strategy, it is important to audit progress and act upon audit findings. An audit of compliance with the trust falls strategy and use of documentation was undertaken in September 2003 by the trust clinical effectiveness team. Findings at the time highlighted patchy use of documentation within the trust and varying levels of knowledge of policies and assessment processes, with the most senior grades of nursing staff having the most knowledge. This was worrying because it was recognized that the less senior grades of staff (D and E grades at the time of the audit) were more likely to undertake the assessment. A key action following this audit was for 'falls champions' to feed back results to their individual directorate, increase monitoring of adherence to the trust falls strategy and examine methods of delivering education.

While acknowledging the challenges in relation to older people who fall in hospital and recognizing the areas for development as identified in recent audits, there is nevertheless a clear strategic approach to falls within this acute trust that has been driven by a core group of staff committed to meeting the National Service Framework targets of reducing both the number of falls and their adverse consequences.

In focusing on these developments it is important that the reader is clear that there is currently no consistent evidence for the prevention of falls in hospital (Chang et al. 2004). Furthermore, the recent NICE guidelines (NICE 2004) do not cover the prevention of falls in acute settings. However, the evidence base relating to falls prevention in hospitals is increasing, with some positive results (Haines et al. 2004, Healey et al. 2004), and as it improves we can strive to reduce the number of falls and falls-related injuries that occur in hospital.

As previously suggested, multi-professional team working and multiple intervention strategies are seen as the most effective means of falls prevention and management. Each member of the team has their own area of expertise, and in order to ensure an effective coordinated approach it is important for there to be good communication between the various team members, patients, relatives and carers. An integral part of discharge planning should include measures to support the patient who is at risk of falling. Physiotherapy staff can assist in problems of gait, balance and posture, including assessment for suitable footwear and walking aids.

Physiotherapy intervention may still be required after discharge home, and referral to appropriate community services will be necessary if this is the case. Occupational therapy input can include an assessment of a patient's suitability for devices that will maintain independence and reduce the risk of falls. A home assessment can be invaluable to a patient who is at risk of falling, with hazards being identified and modified as appropriate. Modification of environmental risk factors is dependent on a patient's compliance and in order to gain the patient's trust it is important to act sensitively when suggesting modifications.

Discharge planning should also include consideration of referral to a community falls service. Patients in our own trust who have fallen twice or more in the previous 6 months are referred to a community falls service. A member of the trust Falls Group provides representation on the district falls group, with particular reference to the development of policies and guidelines. Working collaboratively has resulted in the development of policies and protocols such as foot care advice, side rail and hip protector policies and referral guidelines that are now used in the acute and community trusts.

Conclusion

Falls and falls-related health problems look set to remain a major health care issue for the future. When considering the use of scarce resources in an already overstretched NHS, it is important to ensure that falls prevention and management strategies are based on sound evidence and targeted at those people who will benefit most.

Further work needs to be done in order to understand more fully the role of certain medical, physiological and environmental factors in predisposing older people to falls (Lord et al. 2001). Falls awareness needs to be raised in both acute and community settings, and should be everybody's business. Help the Aged and the National Service Framework websites (see page 197) provide examples of areas of good practice in the prevention and management of falls, and are useful in assisting us to develop strategies in the prevention and management of falls.

As previously highlighted, one of the most serious and much feared consequence of a fall is a fractured neck of femur. As described in Chapter 1, the antecedents of femoral hip fracture are complex. Further research into the prevention and management of falls and the adoption of evidence-based strategies will, it is hoped, contribute to a reduction in the number of hip fractures with all their attendant problems. The impact of this injury and its consequences in terms of personal, health and social care costs will be explored in further chapters.

CHAPTER FOUR

Anatomy and physiology of the hip joint

Although the implementation of falls prevention strategies coupled with better management of osteoporosis will hopefully contribute to a reduction in the number of hip fractures in the future, it is undeniable that significant numbers of older people will still sustain this injury. In caring for this group of patients it is essential for nurses and allied health professionals to have an underpinning knowledge of the anatomy and physiology of the hip joint and the classification of fractures of the hip. This will help them to understand surgical approaches to hip fracture management and enable them to provide appropriate care for individuals who have sustained this injury. The purpose of this chapter is to provide the reader with a basic outline of these topics. There are many excellent textbooks which focus specifically on anatomy and physiology, and the reader is encouraged to consult these in order to gain a deeper knowledge. For convenience, a brief glossary of terms is provided at the end of this chapter.

Anatomy of the hip joint

The hip joint, the largest joint in the body, is a **ball and socket joint** (Fig. 4.1). The femoral head articulates with the acetabulum of the innominate bone. The innominate bone is formed from the ilium, ischium and pubis, each of which contributes to the formation of the acetabulum. The articular surface of the acetabulum is horseshoe shaped. A wedge-shaped fibrocartilage ring known as the **acetabular labrum** surrounds the entire outside of the acetabulum. It deepens the socket to increase the concavity of the acetabulum, enabling it to grasp the head of the femur and maintain stability.

Head of femur

The head of the femur forms approximately two-thirds of a sphere, 4–5 cm in diameter and thickest at its centre. It is covered in **articular cartilage**, except for the **fovea** where the ligament to the head is attached.

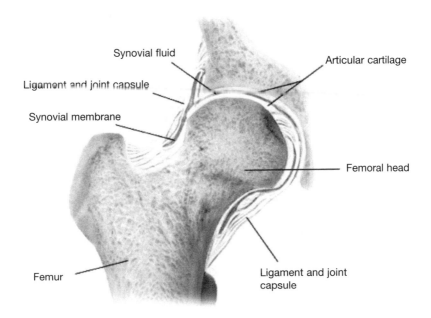

Synovial fluid

Articular cartilage

Ligament and joint capsule

Synovial membrane

Femoral head

Femur

Ligament and joint capsule

Figure 4.1 The hip joint.

Joint capsule

The **joint capsule** is attached to the entire outside of the acetabulum. It blends in with the acetabular labrum and extends above it superiorly. Anteriorly, it covers the whole of the neck of the femur to the intertrochanteric line and posteriorly the neck is covered half way to the intertrochanteric crest. The femoral neck is intracapsular and the greater and lesser trochanters are extracapsular.

Synovial membrane is a thin, highly vascular tissue which lines the joint capsule and covers any structures within the joint not covered by hyaline cartilage. Its principal function is to secrete synovial fluid which fills the joint cavity. The function of the synovial fluid is to lubricate the joint and nourish **hyaline cartilage** which covers the bony articular surfaces. The fluid also contains phagocytic cells which assist in the absorption of microscopic foreign bodies, such as bacteria and broken-down blood cells.

The anterior portion of the joint capsule is reinforced by two strong ligaments:

- The triangular iliofemoral ligament is very strong. The apex is attached to the lower part of the anterior inferior iliac spine and the base to the trochanteric line of the femur. It prevents hip hyperflexion.
- The pubofemoral ligament is also triangular. The base is attached to the

anterior aspect of the pubic ramus and passes to the anterior surface of the intertrochanteric fossa. It limits abduction and extension.

Bands of the iliofemoral and pubofemoral ligaments form a 'Z' on the anterior capsule (Fig. 4.2).

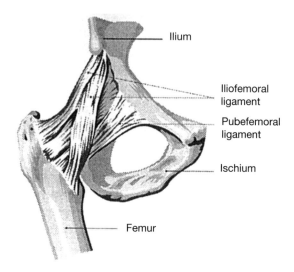

Figure 4.2 Ligaments of the hip joint.

The posterior portion of the joint capsule is reinforced by three ligaments:

- The spiral ischiofemoral ligament. This extends from the ischium below and behind the acetabulum, passing upwards and laterally to attach to the greater trochanter anterior and deep to the iliofemoral ligament (see Fig. 4.2).
- The triangular ligament of the head of the femur. This arises from the pit in the head of the femur and attaches each side of the acetabular notch, blending with the transverse ligament. It contributes to the vascular supply to the head of the femur.
- The transverse ligament of the acetabulum. This bridges the acetabular notch, converting it into a **foramen** through which vessels and nerves enter a joint.

Muscles acting on the hip joint

There are many muscles acting on the hip joint, several of which have more than one action, for example, the pectineus, which contributes to flexion and adduction. The muscle groups form a ring around the hip joint, with

Table 4.1 Major muscles acting on the hip joint

Muscle	Origin	Insertion	Innervation
The flexors			
Iliopsoas (comprising the iliacus and psoas)			
Iliacus	Iliac fossa	Lesser trochanter of femur	Femoral nerve
Psoas major	12th thoracic and all lumbar vertebra	Lesser trochanter of femur	Branches from the lumbar plexus
Rectus femoris	Above acetabulum	Through the quadriceps tendon through the patella and patellar ligament into the tubercle of the tibia	Femoral nerve
Pectineus	Superior pubic ramus	Upper end of the linea aspera of the femur	Femoral nerve
Sartorius	Anterior superior iliac spine	Medial surface of the shaft of the tibia	Femoral nerve
The adductors			
Adductor longus	Body of the pubis	Posterior surface of the shaft of femur	Obturator nerve
Adductor brevis	Inferior pubic rami	Linea aspera	Obturator nerve
Adductor magnus	Inferior pubic rami, ischium and ischial tuberosity	Most of the linea alba, into a tendon which inserts into the adductor tubercle	Obturator nerve
The abductors			
Gluteus medius	Outer surface of the ilium	Greater trochanter	Superior gluteal nerve
Gluteus minimus	Between middle and inferior gluteal lines	Anterior surface of the greater trochanter	Superior gluteal nerve
Tensor fascia latae	Anterior iliac crest	Iliotibial tract	Superior gluteal nerve

Table 4.1 Major muscles acting on the hip joint (continued)

The extensors

Gluteus maximus	Posterior gluteal line of ilium and crest above and also sacrum and coccyx	Fascia lata and gluteal tuberosity of femur	Inferior gluteal nerve

the flexors lying anteriorly, the adductors medially, the abductors laterally and the extensors posteriorly. The major muscles and their actions are listed in the table above (Table 4.1). It is important to be aware that there is also a number of small muscles responsible for lateral rotation of the hip which include:

- Piriformis
- Obturator internus
- Obturator externus
- Gamellus superior
- Gamellus inferior
- Quadratus femoris

The range of movements that take place at the hip joint are:

- Flexion: bending of the limb at the joint.
- Extension: straightening of the limb at the joint
- Abduction: movement away from the midline of the body.
- Adduction: movement towards the midline of the body.
- Circumduction: combination of all of the above movements moving through a circle.

Blood supply to the femoral head

An understanding of the blood supply to the femoral head (Fig. 4.3) is perhaps the most important aspect of anatomy and physiology that nurses and allied health professionals need to develop when caring for the patient with a hip fracture because, as will become apparent later in this chapter, the blood supply to the femoral head may become interrupted by intracapsular fractures (see 1 on Fig. 4.3).

The main blood supply penetrates the head close to the cartilage margin (2 on Fig. 4.3). This arises from an intracapsular arterial ring (3 on Fig. 4.3) located at the base of the femoral neck formed by the ascending branch of the lateral circumflex artery anteriorly (4 on Fig. 4.3) and a large

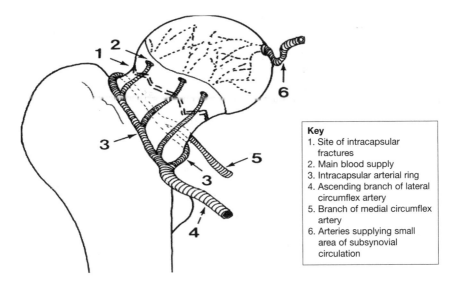

Key
1. Site of intracapsular fractures
2. Main blood supply
3. Intracapsular arterial ring
4. Ascending branch of lateral circumflex artery
5. Branch of medial circumflex artery
6. Arteries supplying small area of subsynovial circulation

Figure 4.3 The blood supply to the femoral head. Source: McCrae R (1981) Practical Fracture Treatment.

branch of the medial circumflex artery posteriorly (5 on Fig 4.3). The ascending cervical branches from the extracapsular ring divide into the anterior, posterior, medial and lateral retinacular arteries at the point in the joint capsule where the articular cartilage demarcates the head from neck. It is the lateral retinacular artery that provides most of the blood supply to the femoral head and neck. Arteries through the ligamentum teres constantly supply a small area of the subsynovial circulation (6 on Fig. 4.3) (McCrae 1983).

Fracture classification

Knowledge of the anatomy and physiology of the hip joint is essential in order to understand fracture classification and treatment options in the management of femoral neck fractures. It has been argued that fracture of the neck of femur is unique for its anatomic characteristics which render the fractured hip vulnerable to a number of complications (Anwar 1999). According to Anwar, the key features are:

- The intracapsular portion of the joint capsule has almost no cambium layer (inner layer of the periosteum) in its fibrous covering to aid peripheral callus formation, so healing in the femoral area is dependent on **endosteal** union alone.

- If fracture fragments are not carefully impacted, synovial fluid can lyse blood clot formation, thus destroying another method of secondary healing by preventing the formation of cells and scaffolding that would allow for vascular invasion of the femoral head.
- The small area of the subsynovial circulation supplied by the arteries through the ligamentum teres is often inadequate to take over the major nourishment of the femoral head following a displaced fracture if all other sources of supply are interrupted.
- The close proximity of the retinacular arteries to bone puts them at risk of injury in any fracture of the femoral neck.

Femoral neck fracture was first identified by Ambrose Paré (1517–1590), an eminent French surgeon, but it was the nineteenth-century English surgeon Sir Astley Cooper who provided the first clear classification of hip fractures and dislocation about the hip (Cooper 1822).

Contemporary practice is to differentiate hip fractures into two broad groups, intracapsular and extracapsular (Fig. 4.4).

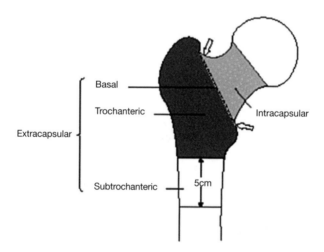

Figure 4.4 Classification of fractures of the proximal femur. Source: SIGN Guidelines (2002). Reproduced with kind permission of The Scottish Intercollegiate Guidelines Network.

Intracapsular fractures

Intracapsular fractures are those which can be identified as being proximal to the attachment of the joint capsule. In these fractures the proximal fragment often loses part of its blood supply, which can lead to avascular necrosis, non-union or both. Because the fracture lies within the joint capsule, blood is contained within it, resulting in a rise in intracapsular pressure which causes further damage to the femoral head. It also prevents visible bruising because blood cannot reach the subcutaneous tissues (Dandy and Edwards 1998). Intracapsular fractures have been classified by Garden (1961) into four distinct grades (Fig. 4.5):

- Grade I: Incomplete or impacted fracture, in which the trabeculae of the inferior neck are still intact. The femoral head is tilted in a posterio-lasteral direction, causing **valgus** angulation at the fracture.
- Grade II: Complete fracture without displacement. The weight-bearing trabeculae arc interrupted by a fracture line across the entire femoral neck. It is distinguished from an impacted fracture by slight **varus** deformity.
- Grade III: Complete fracture with partial displacement. Frequently there is shortening and external rotation of the distal fragment. The **trabecular** pattern of the femoral head does not line up with those of the acetabulum, demonstrating incomplete displacement between the femoral fragments.
- Grade IV: Complete fracture with full displacement. There is no continuity between proximal and distal fragments.

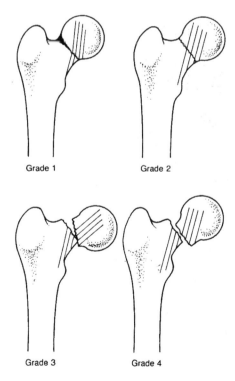

Grade 1   Grade 2

Grade 3   Grade 4

Figure 4.5 Garden's fracture classification. Source: Parker and Pryor (1993) Handbook of Hip Fracture Surgery. Reproduced with kind permission of Elsevier Oxford University Press.

This and other classification systems are still commonly discussed in the literature, but it is important to recognize that they provide little more value in predicting healing complications than a simple system which differentiates between undisplaced and displaced fractures (Parker and Pryor 1993, Blundell et al. 1998). According to this system undisplaced fractures are subdivided into impacted and minimally displaced fractures:

- Impacted fractures are those in which there is distortion of normal bone architecture due to compression of the bone without separation of the fracture surfaces.
- In minimally displaced fractures there is evidence of fracture surfaces just beginning to displace.

Treatment options in the management of intracapsular fractures

Before determining the best treatment option for patients with any hip fracture many factors such as patient age, patient choice and co-morbidities need to be taken into consideration, as all of these will have an impact upon treatment decisions. It is therefore important to keep these factors in mind as we identify the various treatment options, recognizing that all decisions are made on the basis of the individual patient's needs. We should also acknowledge the fact that the treatment of intracapsular fractures is controversial within the field of orthopaedics, with little good evidence clearly supporting one option over another (SIGN 2002, Chilov et al. 2003).

For most patients with undisplaced or minimally displaced fractures, the preferred treatment option is internal fixation with the aim of preventing fracture displacement. In a few patients the decision will be made not to undertake surgery, with bed rest and gentle mobilization strategies being used. This is for those patients who have impacted fractures. There is a high risk of fracture displacement with this management method, and it is therefore only occasionally used nowadays. Careful explanation of the rationale for this decision, including the potential complications, must be given to the patient, and it is essential that regular radiographic follow-up is undertaken to ensure that if the fracture shows signs of displacement surgical intervention can take place.

Evidence to date suggests that the best method for internal fixation of intracapsular fractures involves inserting multiple parallel screws within the femoral head and neck, parallel to the longitudinal axis of the femoral neck (Parker and Tagg 2002, Parker and Stockton 2003) (Fig. 4.6). The positioning of the pins or screws is intended to allow impaction of the femoral neck fracture when the patient is weight bearing. Stabilization of the fracture allows weight bearing and walking to commence as early as the first postoperative day.

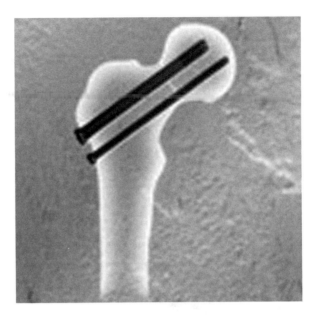

Figure 4.6 Screw fixation.

For some types of fracture, arthroplasty will be considered the most appropriate treatment option (Parker and Pryor 1993). These groups include:

- displaced intracapsular fracture with a significant delay in diagnosis
- displaced intracapsular fracture in a patient with rheumatoid arthritis
- intracapsular fracture secondary to Paget's disease
- intracapsular fracture associated with metabolic bone disease
- intracapsular fracture secondary to malignancy
- hip fracture with co-existent arthritis of the hip.

Different types of implants can be used when the decision for arthroplasty has been made. These fall into three main categories: solid head, bipolar hemiarthroplasty and primary hip replacement

Solid head

Two commonly used types of prosthesis are the Thompson (Figure 4.7) and the Austin Moore. They both have solid heads but can be differentiated by the shape of their stems and the angle of the collar, and the fact that the Austin Moore is un-cemented whereas the Thompson is cemented in place. The rationale for using cement is that it improves bonding and aids stability between the prosthetic stem and the femoral shaft. The use of cement is also considered to increase patient mobility, result in less residual pain and produce a reduced revision rate which might occur in uncemented prosthesis from loosening of the femoral stem (Parker and Gursamy 2004). Cement is not without its risks, however. It is considered to contribute to a more demanding operation and there is an associated risk of cardiac arrhythmia which may lead to cardiopulmonary collapse. The possible complications associated with the use of cement in frail older people with concomitant cardiac and respiratory disease should be carefully considered before surgery.

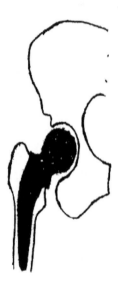

Figure 4.7 Thompson hemiarthroplasty.

Bipolar hemiarthroplasty

The bipolar hemiarthroplasty consists of a metal head (with a stem cemented into the upper femur), which articulates with a plastic more-than-hemispherical cup (Fig. 4.7). On the outside of the plastic cup is a metal shell, which articulates with the acetabulum. It is intended to reduce the risk of acetabular erosion, which has a 20% incidence in long-term survivors of hemiarthroplasty using a solid head implant. Patients selected for bipolar hemiarthroplasty are therefore usually below 65 years of age, because the implant is expected to be in place for a longer period than most other implants. The selection of a bipolar hemiarthroplasty with the same stem as a full total hip replacement also makes conversion easier if required. However, it must be recognized that few patients with acetabular erosion require revision surgery and bipolar hemiarthroplasty is a more expensive and complex operation. The use of this type of implant has to be considered carefully, particularly in light of a recent systematic review which indicated that the role of bipolar prostheses in the management of intracapsular fractures is uncertain (Parker and Gursamy 2004).

Total hip replacement

There is limited indication for this procedure in the primary management of hip fracture, although it may be used in circumstances when there is significant co-existing arthritis.

Displaced intracapsular fractures in the elderly are particularly challenging, and require special consideration. This type of fracture has been described as the unsolved fracture. Before a treatment decision is made, the complications associated with the surgical technique undertaken must be considered carefully (Table 4.2). Any of these complications will have an impact on the future outcome for older people who have undergone surgery. Prosthetic dislocation, sepsis and re-fracture are particularly devastating in terms of their significant contribution to increased mortality and morbidity.

Table 4.2 Complications associated with internal fixation and arthroplasty

Complication	Internal Fixation	Hemiarthroplasty
Non-union	Occurs in 20–30% of elderly patients and accounts for approximately two thirds of re-operation rates.	
Avascular necrosis	Occurs in 10–20% of patients.	
Sepsis	Rare	Occurs in 2–5% of patients
Re-fracture	Rare	Occurs in 2–5% of patients
Dislocation		Occurs in 4% of patients after hemiarthroplasty Occurs in 10% of patients following total hip replacement

Source: Parker MJ, Pryor GA (1993) Handbook of Hip Fracture Surgery. Blackwell Scientific Publications, Oxford. Reproduced with kind permission of Elsevier Oxford University Press.

Extracapsular fractures

Extracapsular fractures occur outside the joint capsule, in the area between the attachment of the joint capsule and a line approximately 5 cm distal to the lesser trochanter. The blood supply to the proximal fragment is not interfered with and there is a greater area of contact between the bony fragments, allowing these fractures to unite easily.

As with intracapsular fractures, there are various classification systems for this type of fracture (Evans 1949, Jensen and Michaelson 1975, Seinheimer

1978, and the AO classification in Blundell et al. 1998). Some confusion also exists with the classification of these fractures when terms such as intertrochanteric and pertrochanteric are used interchangeably. Parker and Pryor (1993) have suggested that in order to reduce this confusion the terms trochanteric and subtrochanteric should be used until a universal classification system is developed. They go on to suggest that trochanteric fractures can be subdivided according to Jensen's classification (Fig. 4.8) into types 1 and 2 which are stable and types 3, 4 and 5 which are considered to be comminuted or unstable. Subtrochanteric fractures occur infrequently and can be subdivided into undisplaced, two-part and comminuted.

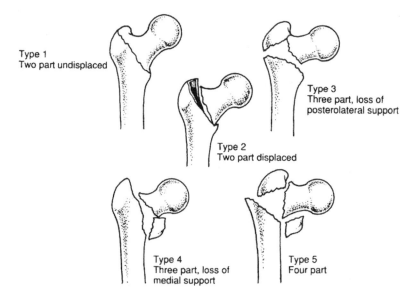

Figure 4.8 Jensen fracture classification. Source: Parker and Pryor (1993) Handbook of hip fracture surgery. Reproduced with kind permission of Elsevier Oxford University Press.

Treatment options in the management of extracapsular fractures

Surgical fixation will be undertaken in most patients who sustain extracapsular fractures. The type of implant to be used in the fixation of these fractures remains controversial. A detailed consideration of these implant methods and the debate surrounding their various applications is beyond the scope of this chapter; comparisons that have been made within the context of randomized trials are summarized in a recent Cochrane review (Parker and Handoll 2003a). It is suggested that extramedullary fixed angle plates, blade plates or condylar plates for hip fracture can no longer be justified (Chinoy and Parker 1999, Parker and Handoll 2003b).

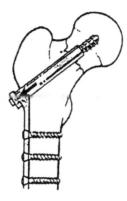

Figure 4.9 Dynamic hip screw.

The dynamic hip screw (sliding hip screw) (Fig. 4.9) remains the most common choice of implant for extracapsular fractures. This type of fixation device has been subject to a number of modifications over recent years, although none of the new variations (e.g. the Medoff plate, Lunsjo et al. 2001) has as yet been shown in randomized controlled trials to be better than a standard dynamic hip screw, and it is suggested that they all need further evaluation before any recommendations can be made for their use (Parker and Handoll 2003b). Dynamic hip screws are not designed to hold the head and neck segments firm, but allow the muscle forces across the hip joint to pull the fracture fragments together until good bony resistance is encountered. Limited collapse at the fracture site as the bone heals is allowed with this type of fixation. This can, however, be problematic with subtrochanteric fractures, because as the fracture line becomes more distal, the dynamic hip screw no longer acts as a dynamic implant but as a static implant with the increased risks of delayed fracture healing, non-union, plate breakage and cut-out. In view of this, many surgeons choose to treat subtrochanteric fractures with an intramedullary nail. Intramedullary nails such as the Gamma nail are inserted via the greater trochanter into the intramedullary canal of the femur. Cross screws are then pushed through the nail into the femoral head and neck.

Conservative and non-operative management

Conservative management

As surgical and anaesthetic techniques have improved, most patients who sustain a hip fracture will undergo surgical fixation. This will enable early mobilization and assist in the prevention of complications associated with bed rest. In rare circumstances, such as when a person refuses consent for surgery, the fracture must be managed conservatively. The aim of the treatment is to maintain bony alignment and ensure that the patient will be able to mobilize once the fracture has healed. In order to maintain bony alignment the patient will need to have a period of bed rest (which will be determined by the rate of fracture union according to regular radiography of the hip joint) and traction will be applied. The specifics of the application and maintenance of traction are beyond the scope of this book. It is, however, important to note the enormous challenges of caring for a frail older person who has opted for conservative treatment. It is essential that the patient is aware of the potential complications associated with prolonged bed rest, which include breakdown in tissue viability, loss of muscle strength, chest infection and deep-vein thrombosis. Medical, nursing and allied health professionals must be particularly vigilant in their delivery of patient care in order to reduce the risk of these potential complications.

Non-operative management

As pointed out in Chapter 1, hip fracture brings with it significant risks in terms of mortality and morbidity. High mortality rates are usually related to the fact that many patients who present with this injury have significant co-morbidities. Surgical fixation and early mobilization can do much to reduce the risk of the thromboembolic and other complications that are associated with bed rest.

There are, however, a very small number of patients who on admission to a ward may not be expected to survive more than a few days. In these circumstances, a decision may be made not to operate. Such a decision will be made in consultation with the patient, family and/or carers, and following joint assessment by the orthopaedic surgeon, the elderly-care physician and a senior anaesthetist. Staff involved in the care of such patients must be fully aware of the plan of care, and it is important to ensure that all staff are able to differentiate between conservative and non-operative treatment. As previously mentioned, in the case of conservative treatment – when traction is being used, for example – the goal will always be to take measures to ensure that the bone heals in good alignment so that hip function can return after the fracture heals. This is essential to enable the patient to mobilize once the period of conservative treatment has been completed. When a decision has been made not to operate, the goals of treatment will be different. The limb should be positioned in such a way as to promote optimum comfort to the patient, regular analgesia should be prescribed and administered according to the individual patient's needs, and efforts should be made to prevent any complications associated with bed rest. The patient, family and/or carers will require an enormous amount of support, and skilled nursing care will be essential in order to ensure that the comfort, dignity and privacy of the patient are maintained at all times.

The complexity of the surgical management of femoral neck fracture should never be underestimated. It provides enormous challenges to even the most expert orthopaedic surgeon and skilled postoperative management is essential. As it will become apparent in the following chapters, the challenges continue as the patient with a femoral neck fracture goes on what can only be described as a complex journey of care.

Glossary

Articular cartilage	Material that covers bone inside a joint. It is normally very smooth. Its function is to help the bones glide easily past each other during movement. It also protects underlying bone.
Acetabular labrum	A complete fibrocartilage rim that deepens the articular socket for the head of the femur and consequently stabilizes the hip joint.
Ball and socket joint	A freely moving joint in which a sphere on the head of one bone fits into a rounded cavity in the other bone.
Endosteal	The inside surface of the bones which border the bone marrow cavity.
Foramen	A natural opening or perforation through a bone or membranous structure.
Fovea	Pit-like landmark.
Hyaline cartilage	Translucent cartilage that protects the underlying subchondral bone by distributing large loads, maintaining low contact stresses and reducing friction at the joint.
Joint capsule	A cavity made of accessory ligaments, with synovial fluid inside. This reinforces the synovial membrane.
Trabeculae	Interconnecting rods and plates of bone, filled with marrow and blood vessels.
Valgus	Deformity in which part of a limb is twisted away from the body.
Varus	Deformity in which part of a limb is twisted towards the body.

CHAPTER FIVE

Assessment

The concept of assessment is a central tenet of the National Service Framework for Older People (DH 2001a) and has been described as the cornerstone to establishing the needs of an older person (Ford and McCormack 2000). Assessment must be recognized as a dynamic and ongoing process that should take place at key stages throughout the journey of care.

For the purpose of this chapter, hip fracture will be used as the paradigm to examine the key components of a comprehensive assessment of the older person in an acute hospital care setting. Theories of personhood and person-centred care will also be discussed, as it can be argued that these are key concepts in understanding expert assessment of the older person. Attention will also be drawn to the difficulties that can occur when assessments are incomplete. Osteoporosis and falls assessments have been covered in Chapters 2 and 3 and will not be revisited in this chapter, but it must be recognized that they form an integral part of any assessment of an older person presenting with a hip fracture.

As identified in Chapter 1, femoral neck fracture is a major cause of morbidity and mortality with approximately 30% mortality at 1 year with a consistent decline in ambulatory status and ability to self care in four out of every five patients (Audit Commission 1995, Todd et al. 1995) Because of their often complex needs, it is essential that these patients have a comprehensive assessment that not only includes nursing and medical needs but also focuses on cognitive and functional capacity and the scope for rehabilitation, which are crucial to effective discharge planning.

Once a frail elderly person is admitted to hospital, the quality of initial assessment and the documentation and dissemination of its findings play a pivotal role in the subsequent exploration of their care needs and the available/possible options following their discharge (DH 1995). The skills and knowledge of junior medical staff, nurses and allied health professionals have been identified as being key in the assessment of older people (Taraborrelli et al. 1998). Yet, as Stevenson (1999) has suggested, there are disparities, with staff in care of the elderly and rehabilitation wards being more knowledgeable about the medical, social and continuing care needs of elderly people than those working on acute or surgical wards. The Audit Commission supports this argument, suggesting that although many of their patients are elderly, staff on orthopaedic wards have not necessarily been trained in the care of elderly people, with the emphasis being on the safe preparation of patients for theatre (Audit Commission 1995, 2000).

What, then, are the potential problems associated with incomplete assessment at the time of admission? For the patient awaiting surgery there can be the unnecessary delay caused by a cancellation because of an undiagnosed medical condition that might not be identified until the day of operation. This can have disastrous consequences, not only in the short term but also in relation to success of internal fixation, rehabilitation and increased morbidity and mortality. Deficiencies in hydration or nutrition which may not have been taken into account at the time of an initial assessment may themselves contribute to delayed operations and may also lead to other serious conditions (Audit Commission 1995, 2000).

Misdiagnosis is another consequence of poor assessment. A patient presenting with an acute confusional state is a good illustration. Acute confusion is a common problem in older people who are admitted to hospital. In the patient with a femoral neck fracture, contributory factors such as pain, dehydration, anaesthesia or medication might cause a person to be temporarily confused. Acute confusion is often not recognized and may be poorly managed by nursing and junior medical staff (Middleton et al. 1999, Young and George 2003). Moreover, in some circumstances the patient might be misdiagnosed as having dementia, leading to inappropriate treatment in the short term and poor discharge planning in the longer term.

Some older people admitted to hospital may be known to have urinary incontinence, but this can be mismanaged in an acute care environment because nursing staff may lack knowledge of the different causes of incontinence and their appropriate treatment and management. Although urinary catheters may be important in some patients who require accurate measurements of fluid input and output, sometimes a catheter is used in preference to more labour-intensive methods of promoting continence. This will have a major impact on the older person who may develop a urinary tract infection and suffer discomfort, loss of independence and dignity. Conversely, when a patient is bed-bound and incontinent they may also suffer discomfort and loss of dignity. It is therefore apparent that assessment must be holistic and focused on the needs of individual patients.

Delays in recovery and discharge can also occur when assessments are incomplete: for example, if patients develop a pressure sore, their length of stay may be increased and their chances of recovery could be significantly reduced. If an appropriate assessment is undertaken factors such as length of time lying on the floor, usual nutritional status, tissue viability and previous level of function will be taken into consideration, informing clinical practice and ensuring that interventions are implemented to assist in the prevention of pressure sores. Plans for rehabilitation and discharge may be compromised if there is insufficient information about previous functional ability and social circumstances.

The above-mentioned factors give us a clue to the complexity of the issues surrounding assessment of the older person admitted to a non-specialist elderly-care environment having sustained a femoral neck fracture. The importance of the skill of the practitioner undertaking an assessment cannot be underestimated, and as this chapter progresses it will become apparent that whatever assessment tool is used it should never replace clinical judgement. For the patient who has sustained a hip fracture it can be extremely frustrating to have to answer a myriad of questions from different professionals, especially when these questions are the same. In an attempt to overcome such difficulties, one of the key components of the single assessment process (DH 2002a) is to ensure that professionals and agencies do not duplicate each other's assessments.

In the acute care setting, professionals need to contribute to assessment in the most effective way, ensuring that information is collected and shared (subject to consent) and avoiding the duplication of assessment. Within the author's own department (an acute trauma unit), the orthogeriatric liaison nursing team undertakes a comprehensive assessment of all hip fracture patients, which includes a falls history, osteoporosis assessment, social history and assessment of previous functional status. This assessment is shared with all members of the multidisciplinary team and has ensured that duplication of assessment is avoided. This avoidance of duplication is a result of the multidisciplinary team members recognizing and acknowledging the clinical judgement and enhanced assessment skills of the orthogeriatric liaison nursing team members. There is a high element of trust between team members and a commitment to sharing information, ensuring that the patient is at the heart of the assessment and care planning process.

When undertaking any assessment it may be necessary in some circumstances to consult other professionals and agencies, such as care coordinators or district nurses, in order to ensure that the picture of the patients' pre-admission status is complete. It is important to gain consent from the patient whenever possible, but it must be acknowledged that there will be circumstances when this is not possible, for instance when the patient has severe cognitive impairment. It is nevertheless important in these situations to obtain as much information as possible from other professionals and agencies in order to ensure that effective and timely responses are made to the patient's future health and care needs.

Having highlighted these salient issues, it is now important to consider the key components of an assessment. For the purposes of this chapter each component will be discussed separately, but it is important to recognize that each component contributes equally to a holistic assessment of an older person.

Pressure sore risk

An older person's skin is subject to the accumulated intrinsic effects of ageing, which include the slowing of epidermal cell growth and cell shrinkage (Marks 1996), stiffening of collagen fibres, and a reduction in the size, number and function of sweat glands (Smoker 1999). One of the many consequences of these changes in the skin is the risk of tissue breakdown, which in a frail older person can begin in as little as 30 minutes after a fall. The human and financial cost of pressure ulcers has been well documented (Cullum et al. 1995, Frank et al. 1999) and in order to minimize these risk factors and prevent the development of pressure sores it is important a pressure ulcer risk assessment is undertaken and actions implemented as a result of the assessment.

Patients at high risk of developing pressure ulcers can be identified using assessment scales such as Waterlow, Braden or Norton (Waterlow 1985 cited in Martin 2000, Braden and Bergstron 1989, Norton 1989) However, evidence for the accuracy of these assessment scales is confusing and is insufficient to recommend one as unambiguously superior to another, or any one scale that is appropriate for use in all care settings (McGough 1999). The Royal College of Nursing and National Institute for Clinical Excellence guidelines recommend that risk assessment scales should only be used as an *aide-mémoire* and should not replace clinical judgement. Nursing staff should also be mindful of further recommendations that suggest that assessment scales should only be used if they have previously been tested in the same specialty (RCN 2001, NICE 2001a).

An informal assessment based on clinical judgement and a sound knowledge of the trigger factors contributing to the development of pressure sores should be undertaken. If trigger factors such as extreme age, acute illness or reduced mobility are identified, than a formal risk assessment should be undertaken. As is apparent from just these three examples, older people with femoral neck fractures will always require formal assessment. Formal assessment should be explicit and systematic, taking into account intrinsic, extrinsic and exacerbating risk factors, and should include inspection of the patient's skin. Findings should be clearly documented, with the score of any risk scale used being recorded. Actions identified by formal assessment to reduce the risk of pressure sore development should also be implemented and formally recorded. Assessment should be ongoing, and re-assessment will be necessary when there is any change in the patient's condition.

The assessment and prevention of pressure ulcers should not be the sole domain of nursing staff. A multidisciplinary education programme will assist in fostering a shared approach and will ensure better understanding of the role of each member of the team in the management of risk assessment and prevention of pressure ulcers.

Nutrition and hydration

Maintaining the nutritional status of patients is considered to be a fundamental aspect of care (DH 2003a). Evidence suggests that in the older independent population 3% of men and 6% of women are undernourished. These figures rise respectively among those in residential and nursing homes to 16% and 15% (Finch et al. 1998). The Audit Commission (2001) also cites studies that have found that up to 40% of patients are admitted to hospital with malnutrition or become malnourished during their hospital stay.

Many factors influence the nutritional status of older people. Four changes in older people which have been identified are (Webb and Copeman 1996):

- skeletal changes
- changes in the immune system
- physical fitness and strength
- fluid balance and renal function.

Changes in the gastrointestinal tract and their potential impact on nutrition have also been highlighted with the suggestion that some of these changes jointly act to cause 'anorexia of ageing' when a person's appetite and food intake are reduced (Gaiballa and Sinclair 1998).

Physiological changes in older people are not the only factors that affect a person's ability to meet their nutritional needs. Nutrition can also be affected by cultural, social, psychological and economic issues, as well as those relating to a person's general state of health. For example, a change in economic status and a lack of access to a selection of shops might restrict the type and variety of food being bought and eaten. Ill-fitting dentures can also restrict the type and texture of food that a person is able to eat, and a person with memory problems might forget to eat.

From the issues discussed, it emerges clearly that older people presenting with a femoral neck fracture are a potentially vulnerable group at risk of undernutrition. Nursing staff must also be alert to the fact that there may be significant variations in older people's nutritional requirements, and screening and assessment should therefore be considered vital (Holmes 2000). An Audit Commission survey of hospitals in England and Wales (2001) revealed that 77% of trusts have a nutritional screening tool in place, with nutritional screening being carried out by nurses. This emphasizes the role of nurses in identifying undernourished patients, and when intervention is required. However, a disappointing result from the same survey was that half of the trusts that did have a screening protocol did not review patients on a weekly basis to ensure that care was adjusted to their changing needs during their stay in hospital. It is important therefore to recognize that 'nutritional state is not a one off situation and clearly needs to be carefully monitored to identify any decline' (Bradley and Rees 2003).

As with pressure ulcer risk assessment, there is a plethora of screening tools to assist in the screening and assessment of patient's nutritional status. The Malnutrition Universal Screening Tool (MUST) is one such tool that is being adopted in many hospitals in the UK. It has been developed for all health care settings and adult patient groups. It has been well validated when compared to other screening tools and is quick and easy to use (Stratton et al. 2004). Again, however, it is important to point out that no nutritional assessment tool should be used as a surrogate for clinical judgement. Screening is the first stage of assessment, but it must be augmented by clinical information which should include the following:

- Does the person have a history of unexplained weight loss?
- Is there infection/trauma/acute illness?
- Condition of skin
- Recent surgery, radiotherapy or cancer chemotherapy
- Multiple drug therapy
- Mental state (depressed, apathetic, alert, inactive)
- Who does the shopping and cooking?
- What does the person usually eat?
- Has the person any difficulties with swallowing?
- State of dentition and oral mucosa.

If nutritional risk is identified, referral should be made to a dietician. Even if this is not necessary, nutritional assessment should be repeated at regular intervals in case of deterioration. Other factors must be taken into consideration and managed: for example, oral hygiene is particularly important in older people, with those wearing dentures being treated with antibiotics and having a vitamin C deficiency being at greater risk of developing oral candidiasis (Paillaud et al. 2004). Oral candidiasis can itself result in mucosal lesions which will have an impact on dietary intake and worsen nutritional status. Attention should also be paid to the risk of dehydration, which may not be recognized because the signs and symptoms may be vague or absent. Problems of dehydration and their impact are more severe in the elderly and a fluid loss of 20% can be fatal (Copeman 1999).

Pain

> We must all die, but if I can save one person from days of torture, that is what I feel is my great and ever new privilege. Pain is a more terrible lord of mankind than even death itself (Schweitzer 1953).

Pain is an individual experience, with many factors influencing what a person might describe as pain, such as previous experience, cultural background, coping strategies, anxiety, fear, depression, disease or surgical prognosis. The experience of pain may be multifactorial and because of this it is not always easy to manage. The assessment and measurement of pain is predominantly a nursing activity, and nurses working with older people need to have the skills and knowledge to manage their patients' pain effectively (Tavener 2002). Whether all nurses have the knowledge and skills is questionable, and there is evidence to suggest a greater need for research into pain measurement for older people.

Nurses hold many beliefs and attitudes about pain and older people, with the greatest myth being that pain is part of the ageing process (Rutledge and Donaldson 1998, Macintyre and Ready 2001). Older people do experience pain, and many of the principles of pain management in older people should be the same as with any other age group, but patients with cognitive impairment or dysphasia present particular challenges (Briggs 2003). This is related to their difficulties in expressing their pain through verbal communication, and can have a detrimental effect on the prescription and administration of analgesia. A study undertaken by Morrison and Siu (2000) revealed that patients with hip fracture and advanced dementia often did not have analgesia prescribed, and that cognitively intact older adults received three times as much postoperative analgesia as those who had dementia. They suggest that the pain experience of cognitively intact people should be used as a surrogate for those with dementia. Other studies have also found that cognitively intact and cognitively impaired older adults experience the same amount of pain, yet the impaired group received less analgesia postoperatively, with the suggestion that it is dangerous to assume that older people perceive pain differently (Bruce and Kopp 2001, AGS 2002).

In the acute setting unrelieved pain can increase the risk of complications that can be life threatening, especially in older people with pre-existing medical conditions. For example, increased cardiovascular demands predispose individuals to myocardial ischaemia or infarction and the gastrointestinal system increases secretions and interstitial fluid but decreases motility, leading to nausea, vomiting, paralytic ileus and bowel oedema (Briggs 2003).

Yet older people can present us with special problems in terms of providing analgesia. Analgesics may not be absorbed or metabolized so well because, for example, of a decrease in liver metabolism. Metabolites of drugs such as morphine are excreted by the kidneys and a decrease in renal function may cause accumulation with repeated doses. Older people are more likely to be receiving more than one drug because of underlying medical problems, and the possibility of drug interactions must be considered.

There are also misconceptions regarding the use of opioids which include lack of tolerance, addiction and respiratory depression in older people (Pasero et al. 1999). These are largely unfounded, but increased sensitivity and longer duration of pain relief are experienced and it is because of these factors that slow titration and regular monitoring are required (AGS 2002). Nursing staff must also be aware of the possible side effects of other forms of analgesia such as traditional non-steroidal anti-inflammatory drugs, which if taken long term can cause a number of upper gastrointestinal side effects, renal impairment and effect haemostasis (NICE 2001b).

Frequent assessment of pain is necessary to identify what the current pain experience means to the patient, and measurement can assist professionals in providing pain relief through pharmacological and non-pharmacological methods. Kamel et al. (2001) demonstrated in their study that the use of a pain assessment tool in mildly cognitively impaired patients was more likely to elicit reports of pain, compared with being asked 'Do you have any pain?' Other studies suggest a visual analogue scale and numeric rating scale are reliable and valid when used as measurement tools to assess pain in older people (Benesh et al. 1997, Rodriguez 2001). However, Bird (2003) in providing us with an excellent evaluation of pain measurement tools (Table 5.1) is more cautious, suggesting that the reliability and validity of pain measurement tools with any patient should not be presumed, and when using a tool to measure pain its limitations should be considered.

Despite the apparent limitations of some pain assessment tools, they can be used as a guide in the assessment of pain and it can be argued that documentation does ensure that pain assessment is formalized. It is, however, important to ensure that nurses use their own observational skills when working with patients and are particularly alert to vocalization and non-verbal expressions of pain when patients are at rest or during movement. Documenting all aspects of pain assessment provides an acknowledgement of its existence, and provides a foundation for effective pain management.

Table 5.1 Pain assessment tools Source: Bird (2003) 'Selection of pain measurement tools' Nursing Standard. 10 December Vol. 18, No. 13, 33–39.

Tool	Use with older patients	Use with patients who are cognitively impaired	Translation and multicultural use
Visual analogue scale	■ Valid tool if self-completion is appropriate ■ Careful instruction and presentation required ■ The nurse can assist completion but bias may be introduced ■ Visual impairment may affect accuracy of results ■ Of the tools discussed here, this is the most sensitive to small changes in pain intensity	■ Low completion rate found in this population ■ Careful instruction and presentation required ■ Nurse can assist completion but bias may be introduced ■ Visual impairment may affect accuracy of results	■ Easily raaeelated as only anchor descriptors and instruction required ■ Successfully used in Italian and French ■ Appropriate for cross-cultural study
Numeric rating scale	■ Appropriate if patient can translate pain into numbers ■ Careful explanation and presentation required ■ Sensitive to intensity changes, but less so than VAS	■ Few in this group could perceive pain as numbers ■ Other tools are more appropriate ■ Verbal administration alone is not enough	■ Appropriate for cross-cultural study as numbers are not subject so translation errors ■ Patient comprehension should be ensured. Can the patient understand pain as a number?
Verbal rating scale	■ Wording requires careful selection ■ Asking how pain has changed since the last assessment may enhance results ■ Not as sensitive as VAS or NRS but too many descriptors can be confusing ■ High completion rates ■ Can be verbally administered	■ High completion rate ■ Can be verbally administered ■ Lacks the sensitivity of other scales	■ Ease of translation depends on target language, but has been successful in Italian ■ Cross-cultural study appropriate once the translation is validated ■ A greater number of descriptors may cause greater error in translation
Faces pain scale	■ Clear instruction and presentation required ■ Visual difficulties can prevent completion ■ High completion rates within this group	■ Low completion rate when modified version used ■ Can be valuable with careful presentation and assessment of patient ability	■ Translation is not required as pictorial ■ Could be used in cross-cultural study but no evidence of this a yet ■ Versatile – usetul where a translated tool is required and not available
McGill pain questionnaire	■ Communication difficulties directly affect completion ■ Shortened version more appropriate if patients cannot tolerate lengthy assessment and ■ Illustrations may assist the patient to understand the descriptors ■ Shortened version more appropriate	■ Validity not confirmed in this patient group	■ Translation complicated due to descriptors ■ A translation may be useful in the target population core validated, but cross-cultural comparison is inappropriate
Brief pain inventory	■ Data suggests limited clinical use but valid tool ■ Shortened version more appropriate if patients cannot tolerate lengthy assessment	■ Difficult to use with this patient pepnatabern ■ Higher degrees of competitive impairment associated with higher rates of non-completion	■ Already used for cross-cultural study as validated in various languages ■ Translated copies could be obtained for self-completion by the patient ■ Could be successfully used by translator
Non-verbal pain measures	■ Selection available but none highly accurate as behavioural interpretation is subjective ■ Checklist of non-verbal pain indicators correlates highly with VRS and may be used together where patient's level of consciousness is likely to change ■ Not completely reliable as behaviour can be interpreted in varying ways	■ No one tool holds particularly high stability in testing but the checklist of non-verbal pain indicators was developed specifically for use with this group	■ Patient comprehension not required but instructions require clear translation ■ DOLOPLUS 2 scale, originally in French, is being validated in other language versions and is the most appropriate for cross-cultural study ■ Pain behaviour varies within cultures and between cultures so caution is advised when interpreting results

It is important that this foundation is built upon and that any patient with a hip fracture receives adequate and appropriate pain relief throughout their hospital stay.

Co-morbidities

Nursing and medical staff need to take account of a person's past medical history. If this information cannot be obtained from the patient, family or carers it is important to contact the GP and/or district nurse, as underlying illnesses may affect anaesthesia and may require further investigation before surgery. For example, if a patient has aortic stenosis a preoperative echocardiogram may be necessary to establish the current degree of stenosis.

A drug history also needs to be taken, with attention being paid not only to prescription drugs, but those that may have been obtained over the counter. A drug history will alert staff to possible contributory factors relating to a fall, and will also assist with information regarding treatment of underlying co-morbidities. It is important to pay attention to vague symptoms, as they may be an indication of problems associated with the use of long-term sedatives or other drugs and could also relate to previously undiagnosed medical problems.

Continence

Nursing staff caring for patients who have sustained a femoral neck fracture will, in their everyday work, come into contact with older people who have continence problems. An assumption made by many nurses is that incontinence is an inevitable part of growing old and as such nothing can be done about it. However, recent national continence guidance suggests that, for many individuals who have continence problems, once the problem is identified, it can be appropriately managed in primary care rather than by referral to specialist continence services (DH 2000c).

Policy initiatives tend to focus on the significant role that nurses working in primary care settings play in the management of continence in older people, but nurses working in acute care environments also need to keep the issue of continence sharply in focus. Knowledge of the possible contributory factors (Boxes 5.1 and 5.2) and types of incontinence (Table 5.2) is essential in order to ensure effective continence management and for the implementation of measures to improve quality (DH 2003).

Box 5.1. Factors that can contribute to functional incontinence
- Deteriorating eyesight: can make it more difficult to find the toilet
- Arthritis: can make moving painful and difficult and may make clothing difficult to manage
- Poor foot health and inappropriate footwear: can impede mobility
- Breathlessness: may make it impossible to reach the toilet in time

- Difficulties in managing clothing
- Toilet facilities may be difficult to reach, e.g. need to climb stairs or go outside

Box 5.2. Factors that can contribute to incontinence in older people
- Physiological changes in the urinary tract which occur as a person gets older
- Neurological disease
- Cognitive difficulties
- Impaired functional ability
- Drug therapy
- Constipation

Table 5.2 Types of incontinence

Urge incontinence	This is the most common type of incontinence in older people. There is a strong urge to pass urine and the person often cannot make it to the bathroom. Urine can leak the instant a person feels the urge to pass it
Genuine stress incontinence	There is an involuntary loss of urine during physical exertion, for example coughing, laughing, sneezing or lifting heavy objects
Voiding difficulties	The quantity of urine exceeds the capacity of the bladder and urine is leaked. A person may feel that the bladder is never fully empty. In other situations a person might feel that the bladder is empty, but dribble and pass urine with little control
Faecal incontinence	

In caring for patients with femoral neck fracture there needs to be a recognition that older people are more susceptible to physiological, pharmacological and psychological risk factors that may impact on incontinence (Malone-Lee 2000) and that functional difficulties such as impaired mobility, poor dexterity and poor eyesight should also be considered in the management of continence (Wilson 2003). Moreover, incontinence is often transient and will often clear when the underlying cause has been removed, for example, when an underlying urinary tract infection has been treated or when the person is no longer acutely confused.

Even if nursing staff have not been specifically trained in continence assessment and management, they should have sufficient knowledge to underpin their practice in assessing continence in acute care settings and implementing measures to meet the individual needs of patients. Assessment of continence should be managed sensitively, because for many older people incontinence is still a taboo subject that they may find difficult to talk about openly. It is important to establish whether continence has previously been assessed, and if so by whom. Contacting primary care colleagues may elicit the information required and save the embarrassment to patients of being asked questions that they have previously answered.

If there has been no previous assessment, it is necessary to obtain information about what factors contribute to incontinence, whether it occurs at specific times and how it is managed. The patient's previous level of continence should inform the plan of care, and nursing staff must be mindful of the fact that containment of incontinence is no longer acceptable without a management plan to address the cause of incontinence (DH 2000c).

Ritualistic practice in the containment of incontinence is therefore not acceptable – for example, the use of pads and pants when a comprehensive assessment has not been undertaken. When pads and pants are used inappropriately, patients are given permission to pass urine on the pad rather than asking for a bed-pan or to go to the toilet. This results in the promotion of incontinence rather than continence. Furthermore, inappropriate use of incontinence pads may be considered as a form of psychological abuse (De Laine et al. 2002).

As with any other assessment, the findings and management should be clearly documented and subject to regular review. This is particularly important in transient causes of incontinence when the underlying cause has been treated and management will change as a result.

So far the focus has been on issues relating to urinary continence. However, it is also important to assess bowel function, particularly in relation to constipation. The causes of constipation are varied and complex, and perhaps no single assessment tool will identify all of them (Eberhardie 2003). In the acute care setting, obtaining a clinical history from the patient will be useful in identifying what the patient perceives as the problem, but this needs to be augmented by more objective tests such as the Bristol stool form scale (Heaton 1999) which has drawings and descriptions of different types of stool recorded on a 7-point scale from very constipated (1) to severe diarrhoea (7). It is useful because of the visual diagram, but it does not assess the frequency and other issues that might account for the stool form and as such needs to be used in conjunction with other assessment parameters in order to assist professionals in identifying the patients' problems and plan care to meet their individual needs.

It is important that continence problems, when identified, are managed appropriately beyond a patient's acute hospital stay. When incontinence persists and has not been previously investigated, referral should be made to an appropriate community professional, such as a district nurse or the continence advisory service, where expert practitioners can work with the individual to investigate the type and cause of incontinence and establish a management plan that will meet the specific needs of the individual. It is not acceptable just to discharge a patient home with a supply of incontinence pads.

Cognitive function

Poor cognitive function is associated with poor outcomes following a hospital stay (Audit Commission 1995, 2000, Hughes 2001). Numerous studies have drawn attention to the problem of acute confusion in hospitalized older people; for example, delirium affects 35–65% of patients after hip fracture repair (Marcantonio et al. 2000). Recognizing this condition and other mental health problems such as depression and acute delirium superimposed on dementia should therefore be considered key skills for nurses involved in the care of patients who have sustained a femoral neck fracture. However, evidence suggests that these conditions are not well recognized and are poorly documented (Fick and Foreman 2000, Young and George 2003).

Our attention is also drawn to difficulties arising from words and terms used, with the suggestion that confusion can be seen in a variety of circumstances when people no longer think with their customary clarity, as in a patient with dementia who may become confused or a delirious patient who has respiratory disease and is hypoxic. It is therefore recommended that the preferred term for acute confusional state is **delirium**, which is defined as 'an organic cerebral syndrome characterized by disturbed consciousness, perception, memory, thinking and behaviour that usually has relatively abrupt onset and a variable and fluctuating course' (Hughes 2001).

Delirium should be formally diagnosed by a medical practitioner and in order to make a diagnosis of delirium, a patient must show each of the following features:

- Disturbance of consciousness, i.e. reduced clarity of awareness of the environment) with reduced ability to focus, sustain or shift attention.
- A change in cognition (such as memory deficit, disorientation, language disturbance) or the development of perceptual disturbance that is not better accounted for by a pre-existing or evolving dementia.

- The disturbance develops over a short period of time (usually hours to days) and tends to fluctuate during the course of the day.
- There is evidence from the history, physical examination or laboratory findings that the disturbance is caused by the direct physiological consequence of a general medical condition.

A diagnosis of delirium can also be made when there is insufficient evidence to support the last criterion, if the clinical presentation is consistent with delirium and the clinical features cannot be attributed to any other diagnosis (APA 1994).

Cognitive assessment should include discussion with family members, carers and significant others who will be able to provide information regarding previous cognitive history. This is essential as it will assist in differentiating between delirium and dementia. A person with dementia will have a history of a degree of cognitive decline over a period of time. It is also important to recognize that some people with dementia will have a superimposed delirium, with evidence of a more pronounced deficit in cognitive function (Fick and Foreman 2000).

It may not always be possible to determine whether a person is cognitively impaired through conversation alone, so a brief cognitive screening is recommended (Schofield and Dewing 2001). However, a small study by the Royal College of Nursing highlighted the fact that some nurses working in acute care settings do not feel that it is their responsibility to screen or assess for cognitive impairment in older people (HA/RCN 2000). This is a worrying finding, as delirium may be the only sign of a more serious and even life-threatening yet treatable condition such as myocardial infarction or chest infection. It may also be a result of inadequate analgesia and undertreated pain (Morrison et al. 2003). Dementia and delirium are also known to increase the risk of mortality in hip fracture patients (Nightingale et al. 2001, Richmond et al. 2003).

The aforementioned factors therefore provide support for the argument that nurses caring for patients with femoral neck fracture should play a role in cognitive assessment and screening. Most cognitive screening and assessment tools can be used by nurses and allied health professionals after some training. The Abbreviated Mental Test Score (Fig. 5.1; Hodkinson 1972) and the Mini Mental State Examination (Folstein et al. 1975) are generally recommended as part of medical and nursing assessments of older people on admission to hospital (Schofield and Dewing 2001). These screening tools will alert staff to the fact that cognitive impairment is present and will also pick up changes when repeated.

When using assessment tools, nursing staff must be aware of timing of assessment and take other factors into consideration. For example, it is not appropriate to attempt to undertake an assessment on someone who

Table 5.3 Abbreviated Mental Test Score. Each question score one point. A score of less than 6 suggests dementia

		Score
1	Age	☐
2	Time to nearest hour	☐
3	An address – for example, 42 West Street – to be repeated by the patient at the end of the test	☐
4	Year	☐
5	Name of hospital, residential institution of home address, depending on where the patient is situated	☐
6	Recognition of two persons – for example, doctor, nurse, home help, etc.	☐
7	Date of birth	☐
8	Date First World War started	☐
9	Name of present monarch	☐
10	Count backwards from 20 to 1	☐
	Total score	☐

Source: Hodkinson HM. Evaluation of a mental test score for assessment of mental impairment in the elderly. Age and Ageing 1972; 1(4): 233–238. Reproduced by permission of Oxford University Press.

appears sleepy or has recently been given opioid analgesia, and the privacy and dignity of the patient should always take utmost priority. It is also important to be aware of other mental health problems that the patient may have, such as depression, and all nurses and allied health professionals should be aware that this may present in many different ways, such as a decline in appetite or a refusal to participate in rehabilitation. It is essential that depression is managed appropriately and treatment instigated as necessary. If an underlying depression is not treated, patients will not reach their full rehabilitation potential.

It is also important to assess the spiritual needs of the patient admitted with a hip fracture. In order to do this, it must be recognized that spirituality is not purely religious but can encompass other factors such as people's search for the meaning of life and the most influential relationships that they have. This aspect of assessment demands a great deal of skill, as it involves enquiry into intimate details of patients' worlds (Govier 2000). When assessing the patients' spiritual needs the practitioner must be able to deal with the answers to the questions that they have posed and be able to recognize their own limitations, making referrals to more appropriate and able professionals as necessary.

For those who have sustained a hip fracture as a result of a fall and who are facing a long period of rehabilitation, fundamental spiritual issues might emerge that might, for example, make them question their very existence as they have previously known it. They might feel that they have lived a long and good life so far, and find it difficult to contemplate a very different life after their injury. They might even question the validity of the life that is now so greatly changed. It is therefore essential that we recognize the spiritual component of an assessment, because in not understanding and attempting to meet the spiritual needs of individuals we may not be able to assist them to function with any future purpose or meaningful identity.

Assessment of an older person with femoral neck fracture should also include previous mobility, functional ability and social circumstances. Each of these factors is explored in greater detail in Chapter 9, but it is important to acknowledge their relevance in the assessment process at this stage because they are all necessary factors in providing a baseline against which rehabilitation goals can be set and discharge planning arrangements can begin.

In attempting to explore the importance of a comprehensive assessment of an older person admitted to a non-specialist elderly-care environment, the individual components of that assessment have been identified. In considering these components separately there is, however, a danger of misleading the reader into thinking that assessment is simplistic and narrowly focused on caring for people in purely physical ways. This clearly should not be the case, and any nurse involved in the assessment of an older person should strive towards a person-centred approach to the assessment process and care delivered as a result of assessment. Indeed it is evident that many of the standards of the National Service Framework for Older People merge with one of the over-riding themes, which is person-centred care. This is a theme which ensures that the needs of the older person, rather than the professionals and organizations who meet these needs are held central (Ford and McCormack 2000).

Theories of personhood and person-centred care have their roots in humanistic philosophy, which places an emphasis on the uniqueness of individuals and their freedom to take a particular course of action through their own personal experience. It is these factors that set humans apart from other species, enabling rational decision-making to occur when competing wants, needs and desires are considered (Ford and McCormack 2000).

Personhood has been described as 'the standing or status bestowed upon one human being by others' (Kitwood 1997). Person-centred care is about getting to know and understand patients, to have knowledge of them as individuals, understanding their ideas, beliefs and lay knowledge (Williams and Grant 1998). It is important to understand that a patient has a biographical history which should be explored in order for professionals to understand that patients have a past, a present and a future. If person-centred care is to be achieved, then key elements need to be considered by practitioners. These are valuing and respecting the person and giving consideration to the person's perspective in terms of meaning and impact and frames of reference (Bush 2003). It is only with this understanding that we can achieve person-centred care, leading to the setting of more realistic goals and outcomes for older people (Hancock 2003).

The concept of person-centred care therefore provides us with a fundamental shift of philosophy in our approach to patient care. It goes beyond the notion of individualized care, encouraging us to respect people for who they are and encouraging us to strive towards ensuring that care and services are compatible with the individual's values. The challenge in clinical practice is ensuring that we move beyond the rhetoric and make person-centred care visible (Nolan 2000). The illustration below will help the reader to recognize how person-centred care can be achieved.

Case study

An elderly man was admitted to the ward with a femoral neck fracture which he sustained after falling off of a deck-chair in his garden. He was a quiet man who had shunned other humans for many years, preferring the company of his dogs. He was unkempt and dirty on admission, and was verbally aggressive towards nursing staff when they attempted to assist him with meeting his personal hygiene needs. He was reluctant to mobilize after his surgery and preferred to stay in bed with the covers over his head. In striving to work towards a truly person-centred approach to care, nursing staff recognized the disruption to the patient's sense of self that occurred as a result of hospitalization. He felt vulnerable and anxious in an environment that forced him to deal with people on a daily basis. This was a situation that he had avoided for many years.

He had chosen not to pay much attention to his personal hygiene needs, and nursing staff grew to respect that he had made this rational choice of his own free will. He slowly began to trust the staff when he realized that they were not trying to impose their values and beliefs upon him and gradually allowed them to assist him with meeting his personal hygiene needs to a standard that he believed to be satisfactory to himself but also ensured that there was no deterioration in tissue viability. As he grew to trust the staff, his biographical details were elicited from him. He had been a gamekeeper for many years and his whole world revolved around his dogs. 'If I could just see my dogs I know I will get going again' was his constant cry. Efforts were made to comply with his wishes; his employers brought in photographs of the dogs, and the dogs were able to visit him in hospital. The effect was extremely positive. He had found a goal – to return home with his dogs – and slowly he began to raise his head from beneath the sheets and begin the process of rehabilitation.

In caring for this patient the nursing staff had moved beyond the simple notion of activities of daily living and caring for this individual in purely physical terms, valuing and respecting him and giving consideration to his perspective demonstrating genuineness, unconditional positive regard and empathetic understanding towards him. They had respected him for who he was and worked with him to set realistic goals and outcomes. The enormous effort required to achieve this level of thought and care cannot be underestimated. Multidisciplinary team meetings were helpful in enabling all members of the team to make a contribution to the care of this patient, highlighting concerns and working together in a determined effort to overcome obstacles to meeting the patient's wishes. The engagement of the infection control team at an early stage was beneficial in assisting staff with concerns about bringing the patient's dogs into visit. The older persons' nurse specialist was in the privileged position of devoting several hours to this patient, encouraging him and using her expert skills to elicit his personal biography from him. As his trust in her grew, a therapeutic relationship developed and they were able to develop mutually agreeable goals. The ward team also worked collaboratively with the older persons' nurse specialist, ensuring that they integrated actions needed to achieve the goals into their daily clinical practice. The nursing team was organized to ensure that the patient did not have to deal with too many different nurses on a day-to-day and shift-to-shift basis, and he was cared for by only a few nurses who identified themselves to him at the beginning of each shift. This enabled the patient to develop trust in those staff working with and caring for him.

The above scenario raises many questions. For example, would this type of care been possible several years ago, and could it have been achieved on another ward? These are difficult questions to answer, but clearly the strong leadership provided by the ward manager and the commitment from all members of the ward and multidisciplinary team in using a person-centred approach to care was of paramount importance. Without these vital components it would not have been possible to achieve person-centred care and the outcome for this patient might have been different.

In the assessment and care planning for an older person who has sustained a femoral neck fracture it is important to recognize that if nurses really believe that older people are persons, there is a moral obligation to work towards a truly person-centred approach to care (Seedhouse 1998). There are, however, many barriers to the provision of person-centred care in the acute hospital environment, including ageist attitudes, routines and rituals, limitations of time, power and organizational structure. It can be argued that in the above scenario all professionals involved in the care of this patient made efforts to overcome such barriers. This should be the standard that we strive towards when assessing and planning the care of all individuals admitted to trauma units with a hip fracture. It is important that they are recognized for their uniqueness as individuals and are not viewed as just another hip fracture. In focusing on a person-centred approach to care, we will make enormous inroads into improving the quality of care that the patient with a hip fracture receives.

CHAPTER SIX

Journey of care

The journey of care for the patient with a femoral neck fracture is a complex one, often made more difficult because many patients sustain their injury in a context of medical, psychological and/or functional frailty. The purpose of this chapter is to provide the reader with knowledge that will assist them in caring for a patient with a femoral neck fracture. Because of the heterogeneity of this patient group and the multiplicity of factors that may impact upon the care that they require, some aspects of care will be expanded further in other chapters.

For the patient with a femoral neck fracture the journey of care begins at the scene of their injury, and factors associated with the cause of injury, ability to summon help and response times will have an impact on their future journey through the health and social care systems and their subsequent discharge domicile. For example, a person who falls and is unable to summon immediate help will be more prone to complications such as dehydration, pressure sores and chest infections as a consequence of lying on the floor for an hour or more. Initial assessment by ambulance personnel provides essential information and assists in building up a picture of the cause of fall, previous medical history, medication details and social circumstances of the injured person. As a result of their initial assessment, highly trained paramedics are able to initiate treatment such as pain relief at the scene of injury.

Accident and emergency department

After assessing for and managing any airway, breathing and circulation problems, further assessment in the accident and emergency department (A&E) should include all relevant medical, nursing and social factors as well as the specific injury sustained. The Royal College of Physicians Report (RCP 1989) which is endorsed by the Scottish Intercollegiate Guidelines Network (SIGN 2002) has produced a number of recommendations for the care of hip fractures in A&E. Recommendations relating specifically to assessment have been discussed in the previous chapter and will not be revisited here.

Adequate and appropriate pain relief is extremely important and should be prescribed and administered according to the needs of individual patients, with the suggestion being that titration of intravenous opioids may offer the best method of pain relief in A&E (SIGN 2002). For some individuals, the use of local nerve blocks may be considered. Of key importance is the need to ensure that analgesia is administered before any painful procedure or transfer, for example transferring a patient from a trolley to an X-ray table in order to obtain radiographic confirmation of a diagnosis of hip fracture.

Initial assessment of patients who arrive in A&E is often undertaken by a nurse, with patients sometimes waiting much longer for a full medical assessment and management plan. The RCP guidelines advise that, because of their vulnerability to pain, confusion, dehydration and pressure sores, hip fracture patients should not spend more than 1 hour in A&E (RCP 1989). Longer waits have been shown to have an adverse effect on outcomes such as length of stay and inpatient mortality (Clague et al. 2002). However, the Audit Commission (2000) reported that although 'fast track' schemes exist in 75% of A&E departments throughout the country, only 7% of hip fracture patients in England were admitted to hospital wards from A&E within the recommended 1 hour. Evidence from research studies have also highlighted difficulties in achieving the 1-hour target (Rajmohan 2000, Dinah 2003).

With the dual problems of waiting for a specialist opinion and waiting for a bed, meeting a 1-hour target is extremely difficult. It is also important to recognize that in some patients it is impossible to meet this target, because of concomitant injuries and co-morbidities; assessment and stabilization of the patient will take much longer, and it might be unsafe to attempt to transfer a patient to the ward if they have not been stabilized. In attempting to raise A&E performance as a key objective for government reform of the NHS, a major target is that by December 2004 all patients requiring emergency admission are admitted to a bed in the hospital within 4 hours of arrival at A&E (DH 2001b). The Department of Health has provided checklists on waits for specialist opinion and waits for beds in order to meet the A&E waiting targets (DH 2004), and hospital trusts are striving hard to meet these. In terms of preventing the development of pressure sores and improving the overall experience of the patient's stay it appears that the 4-hour wait is a more realistic one, although at times even this is extremely challenging for those charged with managing patient flow and bed occupancy on a daily basis.

Preoperative management

Once a diagnosis of hip fracture is confirmed and the patient is admitted to the ward, a comprehensive medical, nursing and social assessment should be undertaken. The most important aspect of preoperative management is ensuring that the patient is optimized for surgery and that any delays to surgery are kept to a minimum.

The detrimental effects of delays to surgery are well documented; they include reduced chance of successful internal fixation and rehabilitation, and increased morbidity and mortality (Todd et al. 1995, Hefley et al. 1996). Delays in operative fixation are extremely distressing for patients and their families or carers, and when delays do occur it is important that the patient is kept fully informed of the reason. Expressions of suddenly feeling helpless, thoughts of why the accident occurred and a focus on basic needs such as pain, thirst, hunger and fatigue were distinctive factors highlighted in one study of the experience of hip fracture patients during the preoperative period (Thorkildsen 2000).

A standard of good practice is that all hip fracture patients should be operated on within 24 hours of injury (Audit Commission 1995, 2000, SIGN 2002). In certain circumstances delays may be necessary in order to correct some medical conditions such as heart failure, significant anaemia or poorly controlled diabetes, and for the investigations of left ventricular function, heart murmurs and aortic stenosis where an echocardiogram may be requested by the anaesthetist. In ensuring that the patient is optimized before surgery, electrolyte imbalances and problems with low circulatory volume, which are common in frail elderly people, need to be promptly and appropriately corrected. Oxygen saturation levels should be assessed on admission and supplementary oxygen prescribed and administered where there is evidence of hypoxaemia. In some hip fracture patients hypoxia may persist from admission until 3–5 days postoperatively (Dyson 1988 cited in SIGN 2002, Clayer and Bruckner 2000).

Adequate and appropriate pain relief should continue to be administered as prescribed and according to the needs of individual patients. Traditionally, preoperative traction was used to assist in pain relief and to make subsequent surgery easier. However, evidence – albeit from a small number of studies – suggests that traction before surgery for a hip fracture provides no benefits for pain relief or fracture reduction, and it is no longer recommended (Parker, Handoll, Bhagara 2004). Leg troughs can be used to alleviate heel pressure, and other pressure-relieving aids should be used after assessment and according to the patient's individual needs.

Thromboembolic prophylaxis

For the patient with a hip fracture, surgery-related and patient-related factors contribute significantly to the risk of thromboembolic complications, which are important causes of morbidity and mortality. A number of studies have evaluated prophylactic measures against thromboembolic complications in hip fracture patients, and an in-depth analysis of these studies is beyond the scope of this chapter. It is, however, important that practitioners caring for hip fracture patients understand the prophylactic thromboembolic measures that can be used and are aware of national and local practice guidelines on reducing the risk of thromboembolic complications.

Chemical and mechanical methods of thromboprophylaxis are available, and these have associated advantages and disadvantages that need careful consideration. Chemical agents such as aspirin, unfractionated heparin and low-molecular-weight heparins protect against deep-vein thrombosis in the lower limb (Handoll, Farrar et al. 2004). They are also relatively cheap, easy to administer and can be used outside an acute hospital environment. Disadvantages associated with their use include the risk of haemorrhage both into the wound and into the spinal cord with neuroaxial anaesthesia (Warwick 2004).

Mechanical foot and calf pumping devices have no haemorrhagic side effects or interactions, appear to prevent deep-vein thrombosis and may protect against pulmonary embolism (Handoll, Parker et al. 2004). However, compliance is a major issue with these mechanical devices and they are also impractical beyond the acute hospital environment. There appears to be no evidence for the efficacy of graduated elastic compression stockings in hip fracture patients (PEP Trial 2000).

This risk/benefit ratio of thromboembolic prophylaxis must be carefully calculated, and it is important that prophylactic thromboembolic protocols are clearly established and form an integral part of the care provided for the patient with a femoral neck fracture.

Consent for surgery

Most patients who sustain a femoral neck fracture will require an operation. Before surgery, it is important to obtain informed consent from the patient. It is good practice to obtain written consent if treatment is complex, or involves significant risks or side effects. National guidelines have been published to ensure that when patients consent to examination or treatment, best practice is adopted throughout the NHS (DH 2001c,

2002b). Particular issues that may arise when seeking consent from older people are the focus of a separate booklet (DH 2001d). Obtaining consent for surgery should be seen as part of the process and not a one-off event. For a person's consent to be valid, the person must be:

- capable of taking that particular decision ('competent')
- acting voluntarily (not under pressure or duress from anyone)
- provided with enough information to enable them to make the decision (DH 2001d).

Information provided should include treatment options; the benefits of the options; the risks, if any, of each option; why the operation is thought to be necessary; the risks associated with not having surgery; and how the patient should expect to feel immediately after the procedure and with reference to future state of health and lifestyle. The patients should be given the time and support necessary to make the decision and should be aware that they are entitled to change their minds or withdraw their consent at any time if they are competent to do so, even if refusal to accept treatment would be detrimental to their health.

In all circumstances it should be assumed that a patient has capacity unless proved otherwise, but some patients with femoral neck fracture may be unable to make decisions regarding surgery – for example, if they have advanced dementia. However, incapacity should not be arbitrarily decided but should be based on an objective assessment of a person's ability to comprehend and use information to make a choice. Orthopaedic surgeons may need to seek the assistance of specialist colleagues in their assessment of the patient. Relatives and/or carers can provide useful information and can be involved in decision-making, but no one can give consent on behalf of adults who are not capable of giving consent for themselves. In legal terms, it is the responsibility of the health professional responsible for the patient's care to decide whether or not a particular treatment is in that patient's best interest.

Consent is an extremely important aspect of clinical governance, which ensures that patients receive high-quality and safe care, and it is important that nurses and allied health professionals are aware of the key issues relating to informed consent, voluntary decision-making and 'best interest' decisions when patients no longer have capacity.

Preoperative fasting

In preparation for surgery, it is a medical and legal requirement that a patient must not be anaesthetized without a period of fasting from food and fluids, except in the case of emergency surgery (Hung 1992). Preoperative fasting is necessary in order to minimize the risk, in the absence of a gag reflex, of the patient inhaling gastric contents while under anaesthetic (Rodgers 2000). Several studies have demonstrated that it is safe practice for patients to receive food for up to 6–8 hours before surgery (Chapman 1996, Jester and Williams 1999) and clear fluids 2–4 hours before anaesthesia (Phillips et al. 1993, Gilbert et al. 1995). During preoperative fasting the body will draw on its own reserves and enter a period of catabolism that can have a detrimental effect, leaving patients with insufficient strength and energy to enable them to cope with their postoperative recovery (Rodgers 2000, Silk and Menzies Gow 2001). It has been suggested that, despite this growing body of evidence, 'practice appears to be based on custom and tradition and to accommodate the unpredictability of the operation list rather than what is best for the patient' (Watson and Rinomhota 2002). When it is necessary to cancel surgery, ward staff must be informed as early as possible so that the patient can recommence fluid and food intake right away.

Many patients with hip fracture will be taking therapeutic drugs for concurrent diseases, and it has been suggested that concerns about preoperative fasting might be a significant factor in the omission of their usual concurrent drug treatment (Connolly and Cunningham 2000). There is also evidence of inequalities in the prescription and administration of regular medications in the perioperative period (Wyld and Nimmo 1998). However, many therapeutic drugs can be continued right through the perioperative period, with the last dose taken, with a sip of water, up to 2 hours before the procedure and then resumed on recovery (DTB 1999). There are some exceptions, and that is why close liaison with anaesthetic colleagues is important when considering the consequences of continuing or withdrawing drugs perioperatively. Preoperative assessment by medical staff can ensure that such decisions are made in advance of surgery (DTB 1999).

Preoperative preparation of the patient with a hip fracture requires the surgical team, anaesthetists, ward and theatre staff to work collaboratively in order to optimize patient care and outcomes. Psychological as well as physical preparation of the patient is important. Patients need to be kept fully informed about what is happening to them, and the rationale behind the treatment plans should be carefully explained: for example, the reason for supplementary oxygen therapy or administration of intravenous fluids.

Operative stage

As explained in Chapter 4, surgical fixation of a hip fracture is dependent upon the site of the fracture and may involve either fixation of the fracture or replacement of the femoral head with an arthroplasty. Hip fracture surgery represents one of the most common orthopaedic procedures and, because of factors such as co-morbidities and poor quality of bone, requires expert technical skills by surgeons and anaesthetists involved in the patient's care. The Royal College of Physicians recommends that hip fracture operations should be carried out by experienced doctors, but the Scottish Hip Fracture Audit Report (2002) and the Audit Commission (1995) have drawn attention to the variations in the grade and experience of surgeon carrying out hip fracture surgery. A more recent Audit Commission report (2000) indicates that there have been some improvements, with only a few hip fracture operations being carried out by unsupervised senior house officer surgeons. This is not reflected in anaesthetic care, however (Table 6.1), and progress still needs to be made in this area.

Table 6.1 Operations carried out by unsupervised SHOs. Reprinted with kind permission of Her Majesty's Stationers Office.

Operations carried out by unsupervised SHOs, 1999 – surgeons compared with anaesthetists.

Only a few operations are still carried out by unsupervised SHO surgeons, but for anaesthetists there is much more room for improvement.

Percentage of operations carried out by unsupervised SHOs

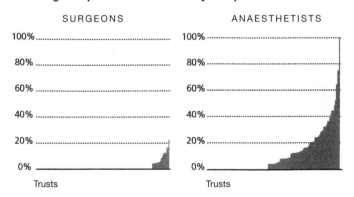

Note: Many trusts reported zero operations carried out by unsupervised SHOs.

Source: Audit Commission Survey 2000.

The most common types of anaesthesia used in the management of hip fractures are **general** and **spinal** anaesthesia. Both types have associated disadvantages, as outlined in Table 6.2. A recent Cochrane review concluded that spinal and general anaesthesia appear to produce comparable results for the outcomes studied. It is further suggested that spinal anaesthesia may reduce short-term mortality, but no conclusion can be drawn for longer-term mortality (Parker, Handoll, Griffiths 2004a). Thus the type of anaesthesia used for hip fracture surgery is determined by the personal preference of the anaesthetist concerned. The decision on what type of anaesthesia to use should be made after consideration of the physiological, pharmacodynamic and pharmokinetic impact of the ageing process and the impact of the surgical pathology itself and any co-existing diseases of the particular patient (Cutfield 2002).

Table 6.2 Potential complications of general and spinal anaesthesia

General	Spinal (regional)
Adverse reaction to drug used	Intraoperative hypotension
Difficulty in establishing an airway	Cerebrovascular ischaemia/infarction
Difficulty in maintaining an airway	Cardiovascular ischaemia/infarction
Intraoperative hypotension	Inadequate regional block
Aspiration of gastric contents	Damage to local structures
Postoperative nausea	Headache secondary to leakage of cerebrospinal fluid from the dural puncture site
Respiratory depression	
Damage to teeth	
Damage to upper airways	

Antibiotic prophylaxis for the patient with a hip fracture has been demonstrated to be effective in reducing nosocomial infection after hip surgery and should be offered to those undergoing surgery for closed fracture fixation (Gillespie and Walenkamp 2004).

As illustrated above, the journey of care from the time of the accident to surgical fixation of a hip fracture is much more complicated than it first appears when 'yet another hip fracture' is admitted to the ward. It is important that nurses and allied health professionals are aware of the potential difficulties that individual patients might experience during this first stage of the journey. Factors relating to the immediate postoperative care of the patient will now be considered, and again the picture presented will demonstrate the complex challenges that face professionals caring for any patient who has sustained a femoral neck fracture.

Early postoperative management

The early postoperative management of the patient with a hip fracture should focus on pain relief, the monitoring of vital signs and fluid input/output balance.

Pain relief

As with the preoperative stage of care, it is essential that patients in the early postoperative period and indeed throughout their stay receive adequate and appropriate pain relief that meets their individual needs. Regular assessment and charting of pain scores have been discussed in Chapter 5. The provision of adequate and appropriate pain relief for postoperative patients is associated with reduced cardiovascular, respiratory and gastrointestinal morbidity and is thought to enhance early mobilization (SIGN 2002).

Monitoring of vital signs

Monitoring of vital signs is an essential component of the postoperative care of a patient, and healthcare workers should be competent in undertaking a systematic and comprehensive approach to patient assessment to enable the early recognition of potential or actual deterioration in the patient's condition (DH 2003a). For many patients with a hip fracture the postoperative recovery period will be an uneventful one, but nursing staff must be alert to the risk of potential or actual deterioration in the patient's condition. Postoperative observations of the patient should include pulse, blood pressure, temperature, respiratory rate, oxygen saturation levels, and fluid intake and output measurements. Respiratory rate, heart rate and the adequacy of oxygenation are the most important physiological indicators of patients who are becoming critically ill in the ward environment (McArthur-Rouse 2001).

Over recent years several physiological scoring systems such as the Modified Early Warning System (MEWS) (DH 2003b) have been developed to assist healthcare workers to recognize and treat patients who become acutely ill in the ward environment. Courses such as Acute Life Threatening Events Recognition and Treatment (ALERT) use a highly structured and prioritized system of management (Ahern and Philpot 2002). The ALERT system (Smith 2000) follows a physical hierarchy that emphasizes the importance of achieving stability in each of the elements in a systematic order (Box 6.1).

Box 6.1. The ALERT system: A–C

A Airway assessment: It is important to ensure that the airway remains patent and that partial or total obstruction does not occur. Functioning suction equipment should be readily available for use in the postoperative period. Once an assessment of the airway has established that it is patent, it is safe to move on to an assessment of breathing.

B Breathing: Respiratory rate, depth and the ease of respiration should be measured. A patient's respiratory rate is the most sensitive observation for detecting any deterioration in condition (Goldhill et al. 1999). The normal rate is between 12 and 18 breaths per minute (Ahern and Philpot 2002). It is also important to note the extent of chest movement and whether accessory muscles of respiration are being used. In such circumstances urgent medical help should be summoned, as these are key indicators of increased respiratory effort and difficulty in breathing. It is important that supplementary oxygen is given as prescribed and according to the patient's oxygen saturation levels in the postoperative period. The provision of supplementary oxygen does not, however, completely prevent episodic desaturation or hypoxaemia in the postoperative period (Rosenberg et al. 1992) but does increase the mean oxygen saturation. For any patient where there are concerns regarding respiratory compromise, regular blood gas analysis should be undertaken to ensure that appropriate treatment is given – for example, the correct percentage of oxygen is administered.

C Circulation: Assessment of circulation is important in determining adequacy of perfusion of vital organs. Capillary refill time, which can be assessed by pressing the skin on the fingertip for 5 seconds and releasing, is a good indicator of peripheral perfusion. If perfusion is inadequate, the colour will not return to the skin within 2 seconds. Signs such as sweatiness and cool, pale limbs are also indicators of poor peripheral perfusion. Monitoring of heart rate and blood pressure is vital in the postoperative period. Assessment of heart rate should include an assessment of the rate regularity and quality of the pulse. Temperature should also be taken and recorded, because hypovolaemia predisposes to hypothermia. Hypothermia can also be a symptom of bacterial infection and sepsis in acutely ill patients (Ahern and Philpot 2002).

Careful assessment of A, B and C are of particular importance when considering the risk of shock, which may occur in the postoperative stage. Increased heart rate and respiratory rate are two of the earliest signs of shock, with hypotension often being a later sign. If hypotension is left untreated the patient's condition will rapidly deteriorate, and it should therefore always be considered as an acute medical emergency.

There are five different types of shock: hypovolaemic, cardiogenic, neurogenic, anaphylactic and septic (Table 6.3). Each of these produces different signs and symptoms but they will all eventually cause circulatory collapse if left untreated (Collins 2000).

Table 6.3 Types of shock

Type	Description
Hypovolaemic	Due to loss of circulating volume, for example, haemorrhage or dehydration
Cardiogenic	Due to a reduction in the ability of the heart to pump effectively
Neurogenic	Damage or dysfunction of the sympathetic nervous system, resulting in vasodilatation and bradycardia
Septic	Vasodilatation and increased capillary permeability secondary to the release of vasoactive substances
Anaphylactic	Vasodilatation as a result of hypersensitivity to an antigen or allergen

There are three distinct stages of shock, which can be summarized as follows:

- Compensatory: Complex physiological responses occur as the body tries to overcome the shock and preserve life. Nerves and hormones work to protect the body and maintain the blood pressure and volume within normal limits. An example of this is when noradrenaline and adrenaline are released in response to the detection of a lowered blood pressure by the baroreceptors which control blood pressure. As a result, blood pressure and pulse rates are raised in response to the vasoconstriction caused by the release of adrenaline and noradrenaline. There is also vasoconstriction of the skin, kidneys and other organs which ensures that the blood supply is concentrated to the most vital organs, the brain and heart.
- Progression: If the originating problem is not corrected, compensatory mechanisms will begin to fail, making the perfusion of vital organs difficult to maintain. At this stage there may be failure of an organ, and as one organ fails there will inevitably be an effect on other organs, eventually leading to multi-organ failure.
- Refractory: At this stage vital organs have failed and the shock can no longer be reversed. Death is imminent (Smeltzer and Bare 2000).

Shock is an unstable, dynamic state in which the patient's condition either improves or worsens and it is therefore important that nursing staff undertaking postoperative observations have an underpinning knowledge of the stages of shock and are alert to the potential for its occurrence in the postoperative patient. Recognizing and managing the signs and symptoms of shock can substantially increase the patient's chance of survival, and the use of physiological scoring systems can assist greatly in the assessment and management of the patient with a hip fracture both pre- and postoperatively.

Patients with a femoral neck fracture are particularly vulnerable to hypovolaemic shock, which may occur as a result of blood loss at the time of injury or during the operation itself. For patients with pre-existing heart disease and older people in general, there is also the added risk of cardiogenic shock, which is characterized as left ventricular failure of the heart itself, resulting in reduced tissue perfusion and impaired cellular activity (De Jong 1997). There is evidence to suggest that episodes of myocardial ischaemia occur in postoperative patients with known ischaemic heart disease in the early hours of the morning, and are most common on the second postoperative day (Juelsgaard et al. 1998). The use of continuous ECG monitoring should be considered in the postoperative period for those high-risk patients with known ischaemic heart disease, particularly if they have had a previous myocardial infarction.

Accurate fluid intake and output measurements should also be an integral component of early postoperative care. It has been suggested that fluid management in elderly people is often poor and that it should be accorded the same status as drug prescription (NCEPOD 1999). Electrolytes must also be carefully managed because imbalances, particularly hypokalaemia and hyponatraemia, are common in the postoperative period, with elderly women being particularly prone to developing hyponatraemia (Callum et al. 1999).

Fluid balance charts can often be inaccurate because of difficulties in measuring all sources of fluid loss: for example, insensible loss and blood loss, and fluid gained from food such as ice-cream (Campbell 2003). Neverthless, nursing staff should always strive to maintain their accuracy. It is vitally important to record urinary output accurately, as oliguria – described as the ability to pass less than 400 ml or 0.5 ml/kg per hour of urine (Smith 2000) – is an early sign that a patient might be deteriorating. Identifying the cause of oliguria and treating it appropriately is essential if the development of acute renal failure is to be prevented.

Patients who are acutely unwell may require catheterization, but it is important that, if required, a catheter is inserted using a strict aseptic technique, as urethral catheters are known to be the single most important source of hospital-acquired Gram-negative septicaemia (Armitage and Thompson 2003, cited in Redmond et al. 2004). A catheter is necessary in acutely unwell patients in order to measure urine output, monitor accurate fluid balance and, along with other factors such as electrolyte balance, inform fluid replacement. However, it should be removed as soon as possible according to improvement in the patient's condition.

Fluid replacement therapy is often necessary in the postoperative care of patients with a hip fracture, but nursing staff must be aware that there are increased risks of complications relating to fluid replacement in older people and those with pre-existing heart disease (Ahern and Philpot 2002). Fluid replacement therapy should be prescribed after careful assessment of the patient's general medical condition, taking into account cardiac status, circulating volume and electrolyte imbalances. If an oliguric patient who has already been fully fluid resuscitated is given continual fluid challenges there is a risk of pulmonary oedema, which can be life threatening (Armitage and Thompson 2003, cited in Redmond et al. 2004).

The reader should recognize that the A, B, C of postoperative care of the hip fracture patient is extremely important and challenges the skills of the nursing staff caring for the patient. Use of procedures such as MEWS can assist nurses to monitor the patient's physiological observations accurately, and respond appropriately when there is a deviation from the normal parameters (Redmond et al. 2004). Nurses should, at all time, be alert to the potential for deterioration in the condition of the patient who, because of co-morbidities and age-related factors, may be more susceptible to acute deterioration in the postoperative period. The use of systems such as MEWS also assists in ensuring that concerns about deteriorating patients are referred to the appropriate members of the medical team who can then initiate treatment according to problems identified.

Having dealt with the A, B and C of the ALERT system we now move on to consider D and E.

Box 6.2. The ALERT system: D–E

D Disability: The aim is to assess and determine neurological function. It is important to know the person's previous neurological function in order to make an accurate assessment. In the assessment of the post-operative hip fracture patient a simple scoring system such as the AVPU score (ACS 1997) is useful. In this system assessment is made for alertness, responsiveness to voice, responsiveness to pain and unresponsiveness. Deterioration in level of consciousness is common in acutely unwell patients and it is important to consider factors that may affect the patient's neurological status, such as cerebrovascular haemorrhage or infarction, hypoxia, hypoxaemia, hypo- or hyperglycaemia, electrolyte abnormalities such as hypo- or hypernatraemia – particularly if developed over a short time – uraemia, and conditions such as acute renal failure. Nurses must be alert to the increased risk of airway compromise if a patient's level of consciousness deteriorates, and immediate action must be taken to reverse possible causes of deteriorating conscious levels by, for example, correcting electrolyte imbalances.

It is also important to remember that some patients are at risk of developing an acute delirium. The early detection and treatment of any underlying cause of delirium is extremely significant because those who experience even a brief period of postoperative delirium have an increased risk of poor functional recovery (Marcantonio et al. 2000, Zakriya et al. 2004).

E Exposure: The aim is to facilitate complete physical examination. Healthcare professionals should ensure that during any physical assessment the privacy and dignity of the patient is maintained at all times. Physical assessment is necessary to detect any significant factors that may have been overlooked in the A, B, C procedures. For example, it is important to inspect the wound site regularly for signs of blood loss haematomas, inflammation and other signs of infection. Wound swabs should be taken if there is wound exudate, even if the patient is on postoperative antibiotics. This is necessary to ensure that current antibiotics are effective against organisms cultured. All members of the multidisciplinary team should be aware of the particular vulnerability of older and acutely unwell patients to the development of methicillin-resistant *Staphylococcus aureus* (MRSA) and should be particularly vigilant in measures to prevent cross-infection, ensuring that infection control policies are strictly adhered to.

Closed suction drainage systems are often used to drain fluid, particularly blood from surgical wounds, with the aim of reducing the occurrence of wound haematomas and infection. However, a Cochrane review of 21 studies of orthopaedic surgery including hip fracture surgery concluded that there was insufficient evidence from randomized controlled studies to support or refute the routine use of closed suction drainage (Parker and Roberts 2004). If a wound drain is in situ it is important to assess and accurately record the volume of wound drain loss.

Sites of inconspicuous body fluid loss should be assessed, as well as other sites for potential causes of infection, for example intravenous cannula sites. General inspection of the skin is important and should include an assessment of pressure areas and overall tissue viability. Evidence of cellulitis and/or oedema should be documented and reported.

As we have moved through the stages from A to E, the significance of good postoperative care should have become apparent. Once the immediate postoperative phase is completed, it is important for health care professionals to be mindful that there could be possible deterioration in any of the factors highlighted above, and this must be borne in mind as we consider the further management of the patient as the journey of care progresses.

Further postoperative management and care

Throughout the journey of care it is important to ensure that analgesia is effective, particularly before physiotherapy and mobilization. For mobilization to be successful it is also necessary to ensure that underlying health deficits are addressed. For example, if haemoglobin levels are too low, a patient will not have enough blood oxygen-carrying capacity to make exercise viable (Collins 1999). Early mobilization is recommended following surgery and, if the patient's overall medical condition allows, it should be commenced within 24 hours of surgery as this will reduce the risk of complications and promote confidence (Audit Commission 1995, 2000, SIGN 2002). Historically, it has been routine practice for a radiograph to be taken and reviewed before mobilization in order to check the alignment of the prosthesis or fixation of the plate. However, recent research has questioned this practice with reference to internal fixation where image intensification has been used during the operative procedure, suggesting that routine check radiographs are unnecessary unless there is some clinical indication (Haddad et al. 1996, Mohanty et al. 2000). Ultimately the decision for a check radiograph before mobilization rests with the surgeon who has performed the operative procedure, but is essential that delays to mobilization are kept to a minimum with early review of check radiographs if these are undertaken.

Weight-bearing status (Box 6.3) will also depend on the clinical decision of the operating surgeon. Generally, after surgery the aim should be for the patient to be able to fully weight-bear; however, due to bone fragility or difficulty with the fixation of a particular fracture, the patient may need to be partially or wholly non-weight-bearing for a period of time. This can prove extremely challenging for staff who are attempting to rehabilitate the patient, particularly when, for example, a patient has short-term memory problems and is unable to fully understand the concept of partial or non-weight-bearing. Often the patient who is non-weight-bearing will be limited to transferring from bed to chair for the required period, and this can have an affect not only on their physical well-being but also on their psychological well-being.

Box 6.3. Weight-bearing status
- Non-weight-bearing: 0% of body weight
- Touch toe weight-bearing: up to 20% of body weight
- Partial weight-bearing: 20–50% of body weight
- Fully weight-bearing: 100% of body weight

Special precautions need to be taken in the care of the patient who has had a hemiarthroplasty, as one of the potential complications of this particular procedure is the risk of dislocation of the prosthesis. This is because the soft tissue (joint capsule and ligaments) that helps to maintain the femoral head centred in the hip joint has been cut during the replacement of the femoral head, increasing the risk of the new 'ball' part of the joint being forced out of the 'socket' and dislocated after surgery while the soft tissues of the hip heal. Limb positioning in bed is extremely important; the patient should be encouraged to keep the affected leg apart and extended away from the midline of the body. An abduction pillow can be used to assist with this. A good practical technique is to encourage the patient to imagine a line running through the middle of their body which the operated leg should never cross over (Fig. 6.1). Patients should be

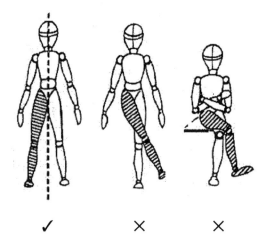

Figure 6.1 Avoiding crossing operated leg over the mid-line of the body: Encourage patients to imagine a line running through the centre of their body and advise them that their operated leg should never cross over this line.

encouraged to sleep on their back and, if comfortable, on their operated side, but not on the un-operated side. When getting out of bed the patient should be got out on the same side that they have been operated on, and they should be got back into bed on the other side. It is important that they are always encouraged to lead with the operated leg (Fig. 6.2). Both the bed and the chair should be at the correct height for transfer, with the bed being no lower than 53 cm (21 inches) and the chair between 43 cm (17 inches) and 53 cm (21 inches) high.

The patient should be discouraged from turning the operated leg inwards or outwards (Fig. 6.3) and should be made aware of the need to keep the operated hip straighter than 90°, whether they are lying, sitting or standing.

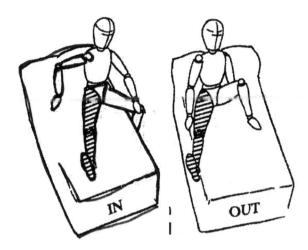

Figure 6.2 Getting in and out of bed.
Encourage patients always to lead with the operated leg. Patients should get out of the bed on the same side they have been operated on. They should get back into bed on the other side from which they got out. When moving up the bed, the patient should be encouraged to keep their operated leg straight and to push with their other leg.

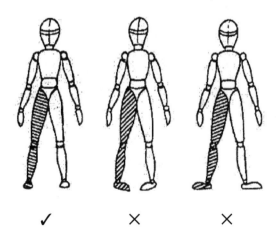

Figure 6.3 Position of the leg.
The feet of patients should always face ahead of them. The operated leg should not be turned inwards or outwards.

All members of the healthcare team should also be fully conversant with how to assist a patient in and out of a chair (see Box 6.4).

Box 6.4. Assisting patients in and out of a chair

Sitting down:

- The operated leg should be put out in front.
- Patients should be encouraged to reach behind for the chair arms.
- The un-operated leg should then be bent slowly and patients should lower themselves slowly into the chair.

Rising from a chair:

- Patients should be encouraged to move their bottom to the edge of the chair.
- The operated leg should be kept straight out in front.
- Weight should be taken on the un-operated leg.
- Patients should be encouraged to push up from the chair, using the chair arms.
- The importance of not using a walking aid to assist with standing should be emphasized: it could increase the risk of falling because it is not fixed to the floor.

Patients will usually start walking with the aid of a zimmer frame, but whatever walking aid is used, the pattern of walking is the same:

- walking aid forward first
- operated leg forward next
- un-operated leg last.

When turning around, patients must not twist the operated leg when bearing weight. As patients' mobility progresses they may need to practise using stairs with the physiotherapist. The pattern for climbing stairs is:

- When stepping up, the un-operated leg leads.
- When stepping down, the operated leg leads.
- The stick or crutch stays with the operated leg.

These routine precautions adopted to assist in the prevention of prosthetic dislocation should be an integral part of the approach to rehabilitation adopted by all members of the multi-professional team in the early postoperative period. Imagine the confusion for the patient if various members of the team use different procedures for transferring the patient from bed to chair.

There are also many hip fracture patients who may not be able to follow instructions or remember what they have been taught. Staff members should be particularly vigilant with these patients, who are at particular risk of dislocation.

Personal hygiene

Patients will need assistance to meet their personal hygiene needs throughout their hospital stay. The amount of assistance required will vary greatly, depending on the individual needs of the patient. It is important to promote independence with this activity where possible, and a washing and dressing assessment undertaken by an occupational therapist may be required before discharge in order to ascertain what equipment is required and what social services input is necessary to ensure that personal hygiene needs are met after discharge.

Pressure area care

Pressure areas are particularly vulnerable to breakdown in older patients. Nursing staff should be particularly vigilant with those patients who have suffered a 'long lie' because of their inability to summon help after a fall. The use of risk assessment tools has been discussed in Chapter 5, but it is important here to emphasize the need to ensure that appropriate pressure-relieving aids are used in the prevention of pressure sores. These should include not only pressure-relieving mattresses, but also cushions when the patient begins to spend longer periods of time in a chair.

Nutrition

As with any other patient group, it is extremely important to meet the nutritional needs of patients with a hip fracture. As suggested in the previous chapter, malnutrition is a common problem in hospital patients, particularly for older people. In some hospitals there is little appreciation of the importance of adequate nutritional care (Manyon-Davis and Bristow 1999, Ellis et al. 2000) although patients who are undernourished are likely to have significantly longer hospital stays and, in the case of acute illness, are more likely to die (Forman 1996, RCP 2002).

Meeting the nutritional needs of patients with a hip fracture can be more complex than it at first appears, and involves many factors that may impact on individual patients. Poor dentition, for example, can affect the food choices that people make, with the greatest effects being among those who are edentulous (Walls et al. 2000) who will be less likely to select food such as raw carrots, apples, oranges, nuts or toast (BNF 2001). Meticulous attention to oral hygiene is important in all older people, because of reduced salivary secretions. If oral hygiene is not performed and oral dryness persists this can result in loss of appetite and poor nutritional status, which in some cases will further exacerbate an underlying malnutrition (Dormenval et al. 1998).

Inadequate nutritional intake may also occur for a number of other reasons, and is often attributable to the disruption of sociocultural, psychological and physiological factors that occurs as a result of illness and/or hospitalization (Holmes 2003). Lack of menu choice, the time that food can be eaten and poor presentation will also have an impact on nutritional intake. Addressing such matters can improve food consumption, and recent initiatives such as protected mealtimes (RCP 2002, HCA 2004) and the 'red tray' (Bradley and Rees 2003) demonstrate an increased awareness of the importance of mealtimes as a means of focusing on the nutritional requirements of patients. The protected mealtimes initiative ensures that disruption at mealtimes is kept to a minimum, with no interruptions due to ward and medicine rounds, for example. As part of a total strategy to improve nutrition in a trauma rehabilitation unit, red trays were used as a visible indicator of vulnerable people who needed help and support from all staff to meet their nutritional needs. An audit showed that the use of this system had transformed nutritional assessment from a paper exercise to a practical tool that enabled patients at risk to be identified and supported with their meals (Bradley and Rees 2003).

Nutritional supplements may be prescribed for patients who are at particular risk of undernutrition. However, the evidence from a number of randomized controlled trials reviewed is very weak, with the strongest evidence being for oral protein and energy feeds (Avenell and Handoll 2004, Milne et al. 2004). Nutrition is a fundamental aspect of patient care and is one of the key features of the Essence of Care benchmarking project (DH 2003a). Nursing staff play a pivotal role in patient feeding, but it must be recognized that meeting the nutritional needs of patients in hospital is the business of all healthcare professionals. It is also important to ensure that families and carers are aware of the importance of nutrition and the role that they can play in helping to meet the nutritional needs of individual patients. They will know the patient's particular likes and dislikes, and can bring in food from home that may tempt the patient to eat. They may even be invited to assist with feeding of the patient if this is necessary, but this should only be encouraged if the patient has no major swallowing difficulties.

Constipation

For patients with a hip fracture the risk of constipation is high. Factors such as the use of opioid analgesia and some other medications, dehydration, decreased fibre in the diet and lack of mobility can all lead to constipation.

Constipation brings with it significant personal costs to the patient including pain, discomfort and the potential for a reduced quality of life if it remains a problem beyond an acute hospital stay. If left untreated, constipation has the potential to lead to the development of serious complications, such as bowel perforation.

Constipation has many causative factors and there is no single method of preventing or treating the condition (Richmond 2003). However, recommendations from the SIGN guidelines include:

- increased fluid intake
- increased fibre in diet
- increased mobility
- laxatives (as recommended in the British National Formulary for drug-induced constipation).

Nursing staff should have a knowledge of the types of laxatives and their actions and must be aware that their use should be limited to short-term therapy, being stopped if at all possible once an increase in fluid and fibre has begun to have an effect. Offering the patient an opportunity to be taken to the toilet instead of using a bedpan or commode can do much to maintain privacy and dignity. Digital rectal examination should only be undertaken according to the Royal College of Nursing guidelines (RCN 2004) and should include a description of the patient's stool. (The Bristol stool form chart in Heaton (1999) may be useful here.) The use of suppositories and microenemas may be necessary in order to soften the stool, but caution should be taken in the prescription and administration of phosphate enemas which have considerable risks associated with their use (Davies 2004). In undertaking digital rectal examination and administrating suppositories and enemas, it is essential to recognize that such procedures are invasive, embarrassing and often painful for patients and attempts should therefore be made to prevent constipation and minimize the need for invasive interventions.

Throughout this chapter the emphasis has been on the physical care needs of patients who have sustained a femoral neck fracture. These care needs must be enhanced by good psychological care using a person-centred approach, which was discussed in detail in Chapter 5 along with an exploration of assessment. Discharge planning, which should commence on the day of admission, is discussed in Chapter 9.

The care of patients with a femoral neck fracture calls upon the skills of health professionals, who need to understand the complex interplay of the many factors that can influence patients throughout their journey of care. Given the number of people admitted to hospital with femoral neck fracture, it could be argued that much of the care that they receive is routine. The danger is, however, that routine care may become mechanistic and as such will not reflect the importance of recognizing the uniqueness of each individual. However, it is important to understand that in an attempt to improve the care and outcomes for this patient group as a whole, efforts can be made to standardize and streamline the care that they receive and some of the methods available to assist us in this endeavour are explored in the following chapter.

CHAPTER SEVEN

Standardizing and streamlining hip fracture care

The previous chapter focused on the journey of care for patients with a femoral neck fracture, a journey of care which – albeit a very smooth one for most patients – can be made more complex because of factors relating to the individual patient or those that occur because of difficulties in service delivery, as for example when surgery is delayed because of operational factors such as lack of theatre capacity. While acknowledging that each patient presenting with a hip fracture is unique, with specific needs, in an effort to improve care delivery and patient outcomes, it is important to standardize the delivery of care in terms of factors such as antibiotic and thromboembolic prophylaxis.

The purpose of this chapter is to describe ways of standardizing and streamlining the care of hip fracture patients, thus ensuring that all patients are optimized before surgery, avoiding any possible delays in surgery and acting in the patient's best interests to minimize the risk of postoperative complications and ensure that the care delivered is of the same high standard for all hip fracture patients.

Fast track admission from A&E

Recommendations regarding the fast tracking of hip fracture patients and difficulties in meeting government targets are discussed in the previous chapter. Efforts to transfer the patient with a fractured neck of femur to the ward area within the shortest possible time should continue, and staff in the accident and emergency (A&E) department should collaborate with their orthopaedic colleagues to look at new ways of working to ensure that any patient with a definitive diagnosis of hip fracture will be transferred to the trauma unit as soon as possible after admission to A&E. As previously discussed, one factor contributing to delays in admitting patients from A&E to ward areas is the wait for a specialist opinion. For patients with a hip fracture, this usually means a requirement to have radiographs reviewed by a member of the orthopaedic medical team before the patient is accepted for admission to a trauma ward. But is it necessary for patients to wait in A&E for an orthopaedic medical opinion? One practical solution to this difficulty could lie in developing the role of A&E emergency nurse practitioners. Comprehensive assessment is imperative to fast-track older people with a hip fracture through A&E and to ensure appropriate referral (Ryan 1996). Experienced A&E nurses are capable of interpreting lower limb radiographs, and with adequate training – which should include knowledge of radiation exposure and risk as well as practical interpretation of radiographs – they could diagnose hip fracture. Combined with a comprehensive assessment, this could contribute to the speeding up of patient transfer from A&E to the ward area.

Practical issues of bed management on any trauma unit should include measures to reduce waits for older people with hip fracture requiring a bed: for example, ensuring that the first bed available is used for a patient with a hip fracture. This may require a thorough overhaul of total bed management throughout the unit, and indeed the entire hospital trust.

Discharge lounges

Government recommendations advocate the use of discharge lounges (DH 2003c) for patients who no longer require the level of care offered on an inpatient ward. Patients who are awaiting medications or transport home can wait in the comfort of a lounge, allowing the bed that has been vacated to be used for acute admissions. Many acute hospitals have now introduced discharge lounges which, if managed well, with a clear operational policy and regular input from pharmacy services, and located in an area of the hospital where there is easy access for ambulances, can reduce pressure on wards and increase capacity. It is important that patients are made aware of the discharge lounge facility, and in the author's own trust the introduction of a 'Leaving Hospital' information booklet has proved useful in assisting in informing patients, families and carers of the possibility of transfer to the discharge lounge while waiting for transport or take-home medications on the day of discharge. The booklet is given at the time of admission, or as soon as the patient's condition allows, and the contents are discussed with the patient and relatives/carers. Written information supplemented by verbal discussions ensures that there a clear understanding of the role of the discharge lounge. Obviously there will be circumstances when transfer to a discharge lounge would not be appropriate, for example, in the case of a patient who is known to have cognitive difficulties and may become disorientated and confused by being placed in another area while waiting to go home.

Clerking pro-forma

It has already been mentioned that a patient with a femoral neck fracture may have co-morbidities that can have an impact on their care and management. There is a danger that these may be overlooked or not given the

	Patient's name (Label if available)
	D.O.B. Hosp. No.

Date: Time: Ward: Consultant:

History (including history or fall or incident):

Frequency of previous falls in last 6 months:

0 [   ]   1 [   ]   > 2 [   ]

Past Medical History:

Drug History: Allergies: ....

1........................   5........................
2........................   6........................
3........................   7........................
4........................   8........................

Social History:

Smoking: Alcohol:

Figure 7.1 Clerking pro-forma.

SYSTEMIC ENQUIRY

CVS: Chest pain   [ ]   Palpitations   [ ]
(Frequency....................) [ ]
        Oedema   Orthopnea   [ ]

RESP: Cough   [ ]   Wheeze   [ ]
     Haemoptysis   [ ]

GI: Weight loss   [ ]   Abdo pain   [ ]
     Altered bowel   [ ]   Constipation   [ ]
     Habit
     Nausea/vomiting   [ ]

GUT: Frequency   [ ]   Nocturia   [ ]
     Incontinence   [ ]

CNS: Syncope   [ ]   Weakness   [ ]
     Dizziness   [ ]   Vision   [ ]

EXAMINATION

CVS: Pulse   BP
     H/S   JVP
     Oedema   Peripheral pulses

Resp: Rate   Added sounds
     Percussion

Abdo:

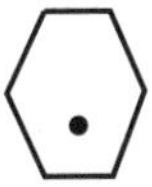

CNS:

Orthopaedic:

Figure 7.1 Clerking pro-forma (continued).

Date: Ward:	Patient's Name (*sticky label if available*) Hospital No: DOB:
MEDICAL CLERK-IN-ACTION PLAN	
Regular Analgesia (*see reverse*)	Antibiotic (*see local practice guidelines*)
Gp + Save (REQUEST AS URGENT)	IV access
FBC / U&E / Glu / bone profile TFT / INR (*if warfarin*) (REQUEST AS URGENT)	Fluids
ECG	Consent
CXR	Mark limb
Aperients (*see reverse*)	Sip feeds (*see reverse*)
Thromboprophylaxis (*see reverse*)	

PRE-OP BLOOD RESULTS		
Hb	Na+	Urea
WCC	K+	Cr
Plats	Gluc	
ECG	CXR	
Admitting Doctor		

SUMMARY	
Problems	
Management Plan	
Signature of Admitting Doctor	Date

Figure 7.1 Clerking pro-forma (continued).

attention necessary to ensure optimization of the patient in the preoperative stage of their care. Orthopaedic surgeons will naturally focus on the hip fracture, but it is necessary to look beyond the fracture if a holistic approach to care is to be delivered. The initial medical clerking of the patient is therefore extremely important, and the standard of clerking can have an impact on the future care of the patient. For example, an inadequate exploration of the cause of the person's fall might result in fixation of the hip fracture but not in the treatment or management of the underlying cause of the fall. Chapter 3 describes the complex aetiology of falls, their prevention and management. It is essential that such information is carefully documented. In order to ensure a more holistic approach to the clerking of patients, it might be worthwhile to consider the introduction of a clerking pro-forma, such as the one that has been introduced in the author's own acute trust (Fig. 7.1) and used in conjunction with an integrated care pathway. Using the clerking pro-forma provides an assurance that all hip fracture patients have a comprehensive systemic review, appropriate investigations initiated and a preoperative action plan. However, as with other tools for the assessment of patients, the clerking pro-forma is designed not to replace clinical judgment but to be used as an *aide-mémoire* to ensure the optimal preoperative assessment and preparation of patients admitted with a hip fracture. A time line for fractured neck of femur is also included, which allows for documentation of delays to surgery and the reasons for them. This is important, as it forms an integral part of audit of the care of hip fracture patients.

Protocols have also been developed that ensure a standardized approach to the management of pain, prevention of deep-vein thrombosis, bowel intervention, nutritional support, bone protection and the assessment and management of falls (Box 7.1). These protocols are driven by current best evidence and follow national guidelines when these are available. This is important, because the performance of individual units and hospital trusts can then be measured and reviewed against the guidelines that have been developed. It is also important to ensure that protocols are reviewed and updated as new evidence becomes available.

Box 7.1. Management guidelines

Analgesia

- Pre-op regular paracetamol 1 g four times daily + regular dihydrocodeine 30 mg four times daily (**unless drowsy, mild pain only or poor renal function – creatinine 180 mmol**)
- If mild pain prescribe co-dydramol regularly.

- Review pain control daily. Patients will not all require as much analgesia once positioned comfortably.
- Review and reduce analgesia to paracetamol or co-dydramol as soon as patient comfort allows.
- Avoid NSAIDs in elderly patients or those with renal impairment.

Aperients

- Senna 2 tablets at night.
- Magnesium hydroxide 10 ml twice daily (NB caution in patients with renal failure).

Sip feeds

- If patient is undernourished or is likely to have an inadequate dietary intake, prescribe Ensure plus 1 carton each meal (caution with diabetic patient if BMs are high).

Antibiotics

- Refer to local practice guidelines.

Thromboprophylaxis

- Refer to local practice guidelines.

Lithium carbonate tablets

- If patient is on these tablets when admitted they should be stopped on the day before surgery and re-started after surgery.
- Therapeutic level to he checked one week after re-starting.

Hyponatraemia

- Never give Slow sodium as a routine treatment for hyponatraemia.
- Review medication in particular for thiazides and SSRIs.
- Review IV fluid prescription history.
- Check postural BP if possible.
- Ask for elderly-care assistance urgently if $Na^+ < 128$ mmol.

Review by orthogeriatric liaison team

In accordance with previously highlighted recommendations, all patients admitted to the trauma unit with an isolated, non-metastatic hip fracture are reviewed in the first instance by a member of the orthogeriatric liaison nursing team and subsequently by an elderly-care physician. These reviews usually take place within 24 hours of admission. Management plans are initiated, and where necessary investigations are initiated. The orthogeriatric nursing team ensures that protocols for prescription and administration of analgesia, thromboembolic and antibiotic prophylaxis and osteoporosis management are adhered to. A comprehensive assessment of the contributory causes leading to the fracture is also undertaken.

A–Z of anaesthesia for hip fracture patients

Delays to surgery should be avoided wherever possible, in order to minimize the risk of poor outcomes (Todd et al. 1995, Grimes et al. 2002). However, in certain circumstances it may be necessary to delay surgery in order to optimize the condition of the patient and manage co-morbidities such as heart failure and diabetes mellitus (Audit Commission 1995, 2000, SIGN 2002). In the ward environment junior medical staff are often charged with undertaking an initial assessment and preparing the patient for theatre. Delays to surgery can occur if the patient is not managed well in this early preoperative stage, for example, if electrolyte imbalances are not corrected or if patients who are taking warfarin do not have their INR stabilized. Other dilemmas include knowing when to request an echocardiogram preoperatively.

In recognizing the difficulties experienced by junior doctors and in order to reduce the risk of delays to surgery, an A–Z of anaesthesia for hip fracture (and other urgent trauma cases) has been developed (see appendix to this chapter, pp. 129–34). The guidelines have been developed by a team of experienced consultant and staff-grade anaesthetists in response to concerns raised at a regular monthly meeting held to discuss ways of improving the care and outcomes for patients with hip fracture. The guidelines are extremely comprehensive and cover all aspects of preoperative care, from simple advice regarding the blood tests that need to be undertaken to more complex management issues such as identifying the need for a request for an echocardiogram and management of the patient with atrial fibrillation. Laminated copies of the guidelines are clearly displayed on each of the trauma wards, and a consultant anaesthetist undertakes a training session with regard to the guidelines at all of the junior doctors' induction sessions.

This comprehensive A–Z of anaesthesia for hip fracture patients can do much to assist the junior medical staff in managing patients in the preoperative stage of their journey of care. It is important to note, however, that these guidelines may be overridden by the judgment of the anaesthetist on the day of surgery.

Good liaison between anaesthetists, surgeons and the elderly-care team is essential if patients are to be optimized in the preoperative period, and guidelines such as these can do much to enhance the care of patients with a femoral neck fracture and reduce unnecessary delays to surgery.

Traffic light coding system

Delays to surgery for patients with femoral neck fracture should be avoided if at all possible. The ability to operate within 24 hours of injury in medically well patients is largely related to availability of daily trauma lists, which should include weekend availability. When delay to surgery relates to inadequate facilities or poor organization, ownership of the problem should not just remain with the orthopaedic team but should be highlighted to the trust executive team where solutions to the problem may then be discussed and strategic plans initiated to overcome the difficulties. There are obviously competing demands on theatre availability, but it is important that methods are in place to ensure that delays for patients with a hip fracture are kept to a minimum. Dedicated hip fracture lists are one possible solution to the problem, as are weekend and twilight trauma lists. Initiatives such as these can only be introduced after their impact on the whole system has been examined: for example, will there be enough experienced staff to ensure that the operating lists can be done, and are adequate support services such as radiography available?

In the author's trust a hip fracture special interest group is well established. This group consists of an orthopaedic consultant, elderly-care physician, consultant anaesthetist, trauma nurse specialist and older person's nurse specialist. The main objective of the group is to improve the overall experience of patients with a hip fracture. The development of policies and protocols has been driven by this group. Current evidence on best practice is also shared at the monthly meetings, where the best methods of integrating evidence into clinical practice are discussed. A major focus of the group is on improving times to theatre. One innovative approach to improving access to surgery has been the introduction of a 'traffic light' coding system which is overseen by the trauma nurse specialist after liaison with the elderly-care nurse specialist (Fig. 7.2). The coding system works in the following way:

- red: patient must be put first on the next day list (hopefully < 20% of patients)
- yellow: dedicated slot must be made available and used
- green: patient to take a dedicated slot if available
- blue: medically unfit, when fit to be allocated yellow.

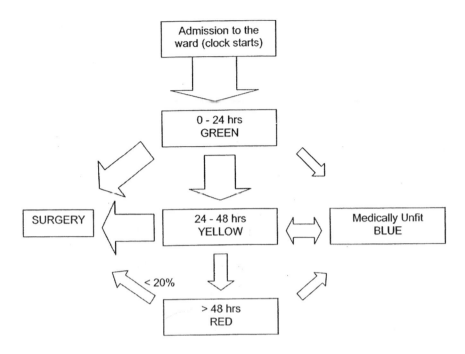

Figure 7.2 Traffic light coding system.

This initiative, along with the other examples cited above, has been supported and endorsed at trust executive level. Regular meetings between the hip fracture special interest group, an executive board representative and colleagues from the local primary care trust have led to better collaboration between the various groups who are involved in the care of people admitted to the acute wards with a hip fracture.

As a result of these meetings, we have established new ways that have enhanced the care of patients with hip fractures. For example, in one intermediate care facility assessments were undertaken by a nurse from that facility before patients were transferred. After discussions with the lead nurse and consultant of the facility, it was agreed that the orthogeriatric liaison nursing team would undertake future assessments. It was envisaged that intermediate care staff could spend more time engaged in the rehabilitation of patients; they would be relieved from the need to undertake a long journey to the acute hospital, duplication of assessment would be avoided and assessment for transfer would be more timely. Better working relationships have also been established with the bed and ward managers of the community hospital. The orthogeriatric liaison team is involved in providing educational sessions for the community hospital staff, and nursing staff from the community hospital have spent time with the orthogeriatric liaison nursing team on the acute trauma unit. In fostering better working relationships and exploring new ways of working there is a demonstrably clear commitment at all levels of the organization and between acute and community care providers to improve the care of the patient with a hip fracture.

Care pathway

NHS trusts are increasingly requiring integrated care pathways (ICPs) to be developed for reasons of finance, bed management and clinical governance. The National Service Framework for Older People (DH 2001a) also promotes the use of ICPs to improve the quality and efficiency of health care for older people. An ICP has been defined as 'a multidisciplinary outline of anticipated care, placed in an appropriate time frame, to help a patient with a specific condition or set of symptoms move progressively through a clinical experience to a positive outcome' (Middleton et al. 2000). Any variation from the anticipated care pathway is recorded, outlining what occurred differently, why, and what was done instead. This ensures that the standardized pathway can be adapted to meet the individual patient's needs.

The evidence suggests that within other healthcare systems the introduction of ICPs for a broad range of conditions, including elective joint arthroplasty (Healey et al. 2002), emergency cardiac (Cannon et al. 2002) and paediatric (Browne et al. 2001) admissions, and the management of fractured neck of femur (Chong et al. 2000), can reduce the length and total costs of acute hospital admissions while maintaining the quality of care. Within the NHS there is similar evidence for some surgical conditions (Sweeney et al. 2002), but not for the management of stroke (Sulch et al. 2000, Kwan and Sandercock 2002).Yet while many acute and primary care trusts throughout England and Wales are developing and using ICPs, there has been little rigorous evaluation of their use (Darer et al. 2002).

Femoral neck fracture is a high-volume, high-cost procedure with a typically well-defined starting point, and therefore seems a good candidate for an ICP. In the author's own trust a care pathway for femoral neck fractures was introduced in November 2000. It was developed by a multidisciplinary team and was based on an extensive literature review, but also incorporated clinical consensus where evidence was lacking. The ICP covers patient care from admission through to discharge or the 12th postoperative day, whichever is sooner. The care pathway was originally designed to start from admission to the A&E department, but this proved impossible, because of disruption in the department's generic documentation and the difficulties in completing additional paperwork during a shortage of nursing staff

(Clancy and Roberts 2000). Our care pathway is similar to ICPs developed for this condition in other hospitals. Clinical care given by medical, nursing, physiotherapy and occupational therapy staff is included and variances are recorded. Criteria for admission to the ICP are:

- The patient must have a definite diagnosis of a fractured neck of femur.
- The fracture must not be pathological (as this would require a different management plan).
- The fracture must be isolated (as rehabilitation needs might be different if there are other fractures that need to be taken into consideration).

Developing and planning the care pathway took several months, and staff education was considered to be the vital link in ensuring its success. In areas where training has gone well, with most staff being introduced to the care pathway document, ICPs are generally well used and appreciated (Johnson et al. 2000). It is also important to recognize that education needs to be ongoing, with the theoretical element of care pathway implementation being supplemented by support given to staff in the ward environment in order to assist them in using the documentation. Ongoing commitment to education is essential, and managers and lead clinicians need to recognize the importance of releasing staff to attend training sessions.

The costs of implementing care pathways are considerable and ongoing, leading to the suggestion that evidence of clinical benefit or cost savings should be mandatory before any individual pathway is adopted (Roberts et al. 2002).

In the author's trust, a multidisciplinary research team has evaluated the effectiveness of implementing a care pathway for femoral neck fracture in older people (Roberts et al. 2004). The study design was a prospective study of patients admitted 12 months before and after implementation of the care pathway. Audit data for corresponding time periods from three nearby orthopaedic units was used to control for secular trends. Evidence from the study demonstrated that the care pathway was associated with improvements in the process and outcomes of this group of patients with complex needs, but also with longer lengths of stay. The process of developing the pathway had benefits: for example, it served as a driving force to reach clinical consensus on protocols for deep-vein thrombosis and antibiotic prophylaxis. This reflects previous evidence that ICPs can improve the process of care in complex clinical cases (Sulch et al. 2002).

Nursing staff and allied health care professionals use the care pathway well and remain committed to it. Although it is often difficult to quantify improvements in quality of care, awareness of patients' needs and the complexity of issues surrounding their condition has grown. Patient assessment and discharge planning has improved. There are fewer wound infections and pressure ulcers, and a trend towards fewer urinary tract infections.

Patients have improved mobility on discharge and fewer have been admitted to institutional care (Roberts et al. 2004). Our own experience is that a care pathway can be a useful tool in raising care standards, but may require additional resources. This has clear implications for those involved in planning and providing the clinical care for this group of patients.

Audit

It is important to examine the care that is delivered to patients with a femoral neck fracture. Femoral neck fracture is increasingly being acknowledged as a tracer condition of interest in assessing the care of elderly people (Audit Commission 1995, 2000, SIGN 2002) and as such is the focus of a great deal of research and clinical audit. It is important that clinical staff are able to differentiate between clinical audit and research. This is not as easy as it may seem, because although they have different purposes, they are similar in many ways: both use systematic processes, defined questions, the same data collection tools, attempts to eliminate bias and attention to detail in data collection (Roe and Webb 1998). A number of definitions to clarify the differences between them can be found in the literature. Put simply, clinical audit aims to establish the extent to which actual clinical practice **compares with** best clinical practice, while clinical research aims to establish **what is** the best clinical practice (Scottish Office 1993). Although these two elements are different, they can feed into each other. The outcome of an audit might, for example, give rise to research questions: 'if the outcomes of audit are not as intended, research can ask why' (Packwood and Kober 1995).

Because of the increased recognition of hip fracture as a tracer condition, a number of audits have already been undertaken which provide a snapshot of service provision, problem identification and improvements that have been made in certain geographical areas. Examples include the East Anglia Hip Fracture Audit (Todd et al. 1995) and the Scottish Hip Fracture Audit (2002). The Standardization of Audit of Hip Fracture in Europe, which was supported by the European Union, was introduced in 1998. This has an agreed standard data set for the audit of hip fracture, with software support. The aim of this initiative is to facilitate Europe-wide comparison of case mix, surgical management, rehabilitation process and outcomes, ensuring the dissemination of best practice in surgery and rehabilitation of hip fracture (Parker et al. 1998).

Audit is also a key component of clinical governance, which has been described as 'a framework through which NHS organizations are accountable for continuously improving the quality of their services and safeguarding high standards by creating an environment in which excellence in clinical care will flourish' (DH 1998a). Thus, in order to ensure excellence in the clinical care of patients with a femoral neck fracture, doctors, nurses and allied health professionals must engage in the multidisciplinary audit of care delivery.

One's first experience of clinical audit can prove daunting. The following information, based on the author's own experience of audit of hip fracture over the past 7 years, may prove helpful. To illustrate the audit cycle and assist readers to familiarize themselves with some of the terminology used in the audit process, the example of time to surgery will be used.

Before undertaking any audit it must be kept clearly in mind that the primary function of clinical audit is to improve patient care by informing health care professionals' understanding of their clinical practice. Essentially, audit is a tool to help you make changes for the better. Also, before undertaking an audit it is important to identify the background, which may require an extensive literature review. In the case of time to theatre there is a large body of evidence highlighting the importance of minimizing delays to surgery and identifying the associated poor outcomes when surgery is delayed.

Having undertaken a literature review and identified the background to the audit, the following steps then need to be taken:

- Identify the problem or objective: The number of patients having hip surgery within 24 hours of admission is less than 50%.
- Agree criteria and set standards: **Criteria** are those aspects of care that you wish to examine: they must be definable, measurable and evidence based. **Standards** are the pre-stated or implicit levels of success that you wish to achieve, in this case:
  - All hip fracture patients should have surgery within 24 hours of admission.
  - All patients admitted with a fractured neck of femur who are medically well should have surgery within 24 hours of admission.
- Measure current practice (audit-data collection): Current practice needs to be measured against the criteria agreed and standards set. In this way we are able to look at the real situation. The time of admission and time of surgery should be documented for all patients admitted with a hip fracture who are medically fit. Reasons for delay to surgery should be identified. The length of time for data collection should also be identified. At the end of the audit period, data should be collated. The initial findings should then be fed back to the directorate management team, orthopaedic consultants, elderly-care physicians, ward staff and the trust's clinical effectiveness team.
- Identify areas for improvement: There is a need to find ways of moving from the real to the ideal, e.g. the introduction of a 'traffic light' system and dedicated hip fracture operating lists.

- Make the necessary changes: Implement a 'traffic light' system and dedicated hip fracture operating lists. Ensure that all members of the team, including anaesthetists, surgeons, and theatre and ward personnel, are aware of these changes. Nominated staff members should be identified to monitor and maintain the system on a daily basis.
- Re-evaluate practice and provide feedback to those providing care: After changes have been implemented, an adequate period of time must be allowed for full implementation. It is then necessary to identify if changes implemented have resulted in meeting the criteria agreed and the standard set. Further initiatives may have to be implemented at this stage and the audit cycle should begin again.

In summary, the audit cycle is continuous but has several key steps that need to be followed, as represented in Fig 7.3.

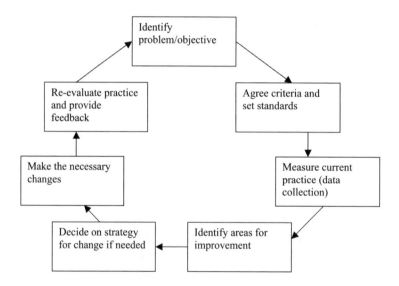

Figure 7.3 The audit cycle.

Any number of factors can be measured using the audit cycle, and the data collected can prove to be extremely useful. Audit is perhaps the most visible form of clinical effectiveness, and in the case of the management and care of patients with femoral neck fracture should form an integral part of clinical practice.

In attempting to streamline and standardize hip fracture care it is important that care delivery is evidence based and that all members of the health care team demonstrate a clear commitment to improving the standard of patient care. This will ultimately lead to an improvement in outcomes for this group of patients, many of whom have multiple pathology and complex discharge planning needs. Chapter 10 focuses on the clinical and government guidelines that have an impact upon the care of the patient with a hip fracture, highlighting why a knowledge of these is essential if we are to progress and improve care delivery to this particular patient group.

Appendix: The A–Z of anaesthesia for hip fracture patients

PLEASE NOTE: These guidelines are designed for elderly trauma patients. They are **not** applicable to patients coming for elective surgery.

- Five consultant anaesthetists and six experienced staff grade anaesthetists who regularly give anaesthetics for trauma lists have prepared this document.
- If you work within these guidelines, patients will usually be accepted for theatre.
- However, the judgement of the anaesthetist on the day overrides anything written here. In particular, if less experienced anaesthetists are working on their own, patients may still be turned down.

Blood tests

All elderly trauma patients need FBC and Coag, U&E, LFT.

- Group and save: all patients with fractured neck of femur, all nailings, major joint replacements or revisions, fractured long bones.
- Cross match: only for patients who are **highly likely** to need blood. We can get blood on G&S in about 15 minutes. If you are not sure, look at the dept guidelines, or ask a surgeon or anaesthetist.

And **also**:
Recheck the U&E as follows:

- Every 48 hours if it was normal on admission.
- Daily if it was abnormal on admission or at any stage.

Chest infections

Chest infection is rarely a reason to cancel a case. Most patients with fractured neck of femur can have a spinal anaesthetic if necessary.

Exceptions to this are:

- Patients with raised INR (more than 1.5) cannot have a spinal.
- Patients with rods or other instrumentation of the spine cannot have a spinal.
- Patients who are too breathless to tolerate lying at about 20° from flat cannot tolerate operation under spinal.
- Patients with known severe aortic stenosis: spinal may not be safe.

Always discuss with an anaesthetist before cancelling a case due to chest infection. Chest infections usually get worse, not better, in the presence of a fractured neck of femur.

Chest X-ray

All patients with fractured neck of femur should have a chest X-ray on arrival. A supine AP film is satisfactory. Anaesthetists particularly value a chest X-ray for the information it gives about the **mediastinal shadow and heart size.** Information about the lungs is less useful because clinical impression is more important than the CXR appearance. A repeat X-ray to assess a chest infection is rarely of any use.

Falls

Anaesthetists are concerned about slow or fast heart rhythms that might cause falls. However, most slow rhythms and fast rhythms are amenable to treatment during an anaesthetic. Unless your patient **clearly** has unexplained syncope, or has syncope with angina, we suggest that 24-hour tapes to investigate falls take place after surgery has been carried out.

We will not usually accept a patient for theatre with a 24 hour tape in place. If they have a tape, we will want to know the result – you need to request the result urgently.

Haemoglobin

We recommend the following guidelines for elderly trauma patients:

- If the haemoglobin is less than 8 g/dl they should be transfused preoperatively. Aim to bring the haemoglobin up to about 9 g/dl and give diuretic cover only if indicated.
- If the haemoglobin is between 8 and 9.9 g/dl, they should **only** be transfused **if** they have significant coronary artery disease.
- Some anaesthetists expect to see a check haemoglobin after transfusion. **Please send a check as soon as possible after the transfusion.**

Heparin

Subcutaneous heparin should be prescribed as in your department guidelines.

Always prescribe enoxaparin (Clexane) to be given at 17:00 or 21:00. This is because we cannot do a spinal anaesthetic within 12 hours of a dose of Clexane. The evening dose allows us to do a spinal at any time during the next day's list.

INR

- The INR should usually be below 2 for most operations.
- For a spinal anaesthetic the INR must be **less than 1.5.**

Two regimes are available for INR reversal:

- **Cautious regime:** Vitamin K slow bolus 1-2 mg IV. Recheck after 6 hours and repeat as required. If more than two doses, consult haematologists. Excess vitamin K may make the patient refractory to oral anticoagulation for 2–3 weeks.
- **Aggressive regime**: Vitamin K 10 mg slow bolus IV. Recheck INR after 6 hours. Probably no benefit in repeating. Consider FFP or beriplex if still elevated.

Reversal of INR is a **balance of risks**. Mortality from fractured neck of femur rises by a factor of around 50% if the patient waits more than 48 hours for surgery. This is due to risks of bed rest and include chest infection, DVT, reduced nutrition, etc. You need **to be sure** that cautious reversal of INR is justified.

- Patients who take warfarin for AF without other complications should usually have aggressive reversal.
- Patients with an artificial heart valve should have either cautious reversal or no active reversal (stop the warfarin and wait). The choice depends on other factors and you should discuss with the elderly care team and/or a cardiologist.
- Patient on warfarin for other reasons – discuss with elderly care team.

Intravenous infusion

All fractured neck of femur patients need an IVI. U&E should be monitored alternate days or daily if abnormal.

Pacemakers

A pacemaker check should usually be requested pre-op, especially if the fall is unexplained.

Diabetes

Detailed guidelines for diabetes are found in the trust-wide diabetes protocol for perioperative care. This is a brief summary. Most trauma patients can eat and drink within 4 hours of surgery and plans for control of diabetes should take this into account.

- Insulin-dependent patients need to be placed first on the operating list. They **usually** need a dextrose and insulin regime started on the morning of surgery.
- Non-insulin dependent patients **do not usually** need a dextrose and insulin regime preoperatively. They should be placed as early as possible on the list, fasted as usual and diabetic tablets omitted. The blood sugar should be monitored 1–2 hourly. If it rises above 11 you should discuss management with the anaesthetist immediately.
- Diet-controlled diabetics **almost never** need a dextrose and insulin regime preoperatively. Their blood sugar should be monitored.

High blood sugars are not usually a reason to delay surgery in urgent trauma patients, unless the patient is ketotic and dehydrated. You should start treatment urgently, however, and discuss what you are doing with the anaesthetist.

ECG

All elderly trauma patients need an ECG. Also:

- all patients over the age of 60
- all patients with hypertension or any other risk factors for coronary artery disease
- all patients with peripheral vascular or cerebrovascular disease
- all patients on 'cardiac' drugs.

Potassium

Potassium level must be > 3 mmol/dl, or the case will be cancelled.

- If the potassium level is between 3 and 3.5, we will accept only if adequate potassium replacement is in progress.

- If the potassium is less than 3.5 there must be a daily check until it comes up and the cause has been stopped/treated.
- Remember you can get an instant potassium from the blood gas machine (take a heparinized venous sample).
- If the patient is elderly or has impaired renal function, please ask an elderly care doctor to help you choose a regime. Also, consider why the potassium is low and treat the cause.

Thyroid function tests

These should always be done on admission in patients on thyroxine. However, if the patient is clinically euthyroid, we will usually accept the patient for theatre without a result.

And finally:

Special anaesthetic review

Please note we will always want to be warned about patients as follows:

- history of difficult intubation
- anyone who can't open their mouth
- anyone with restricted neck movement (e.g. ankylosing spondylitis) or unstable neck (fracture or RA)
- known problems with GA – malignant hyperpyrexia, suxamethonium apnoea, any unplanned ICU admission in the past.

Notes

If your patient has had relevant treatment which is documented in other notes, please ask the ward clerk to get those notes (most commonly cardiac or neuro).

Intensive care bookings

The earlier you book an ICU bed, the better. Please consider:

- BMI over 45
- any history of flail chest
- expected blood loss over 2 litres
- remember there is no HDU facility for orthopaedics – it is ICU or the ward.

Drugs before surgery

It is difficult to give specific guidelines for all drugs. In general anaesthetists should be asked to mark the chart. The following may be useful:

- Patients should always continue beta blockers (rapid withdrawal may be dangerous due to rebound tachycardia).
- Most anaesthetists require ACE inhibitors used for **hypertension** to be **omitted** on the morning of surgery. **But** if they are given for **heart failure**, you must ask the anaesthetist.
- Most 'cardiac' or blood pressure drugs should be given
- Painkillers should be given as required. Anti-inflammatories should be used with care on an empty stomach. It will **always** be OK to give morphine, codeine or similar drugs if the patient is in pain. It will not upset the anaesthetic, and patients should **not** be left in pain.

CHAPTER EIGHT

Developing an orthogeriatric liaison service

Older people admitted to trauma wards have a lot in common with those admitted to elderly-care wards. Their needs are often complex, with many of them experiencing at least one co-morbidity common in old age: Parkinson's disease, dementia, hypertension or heart failure. Timely and appropriate intervention from the elderly-care team (elderly-care physicians and nurses with expertise in the care of older people) can do much to assist in the assessment, perioperative management and rehabilitation of elderly patients with a hip fracture.

Several reports have highlighted key themes in the management of patients with a hip fracture (Audit Commission 1995, Todd et al. 1995, SIGN 2002). One of these is that physicians specializing in care of the elderly should be involved. The National Service Framework for Older People states 'At least one general ward in an acute hospital should be developed as a centre of excellence for orthogeriatric practice' (DH 2001a). It does not, however, recommend a particular orthogeriatric model, suggesting that this should be agreed at local level. Different models for developing orthogeriatric services have been identified:

- The traditional model: Patients with a hip fracture are admitted to a trauma ward and their care and rehabilitation are primarily managed by the orthopaedic consultant and team. In this model support from the elderly-care team is on a consultative basis.
- A variation on the traditional model: Patients are admitted to a trauma ward and there is regular input from the elderly-care team; for example, a twice-weekly multidisciplinary ward round with orthopaedic surgeons and elderly-care physicians.
- Preoperative management by the orthopaedic team with early post-operative transfer to an elderly-care rehabilitation unit: This may involve combined orthopaedic and elderly-care ward rounds in the rehabilitation unit.
- Combined orthogeriatric care: Patients are admitted to a specialist orthogeriatric ward under the care of both elderly-care physicians and orthopaedic surgeons. The patients are assessed by the elderly-care team both pre- and postoperatively (Audit Commission 1995).

All of these models have their strengths and weaknesses, and it must be acknowledged that the choice of model will depend greatly on local resources and the actual numbers of patients requiring orthogeriatric input. However, a recent publication by the British Orthopaedic Association (BOA 2003) has suggested that the combined orthogeriatric care model offers the best opportunity to ensure the highest standard of patient care.

Clearly, when considering the development of an orthogeriatric liaison service these factors need to be taken into account. Of further importance is the need to ensure that any service arrangements are clearly identified and unambiguous. At the earliest stage in the development of the service, somebody needs to be identified to take overall responsibility for all aspects of care, providing an overview and ensuring that all stages in the process of care fit smoothly together.

Orthopaedic surgeons and elderly-care physicians also need to share responsibility for ensuring that procedures, protocols, communication and liaison mechanisms have been established. This will help to ensure that liaison actually happens in practice (SIGN 2002).

The purpose of this chapter is to describe the benefits and pitfalls of developing an orthogeriatric liaison service in a large university teaching hospital.

Establishing the need for a service

Before developing an orthogeriatric liaison service it is important to identify any deficiencies in the existing framework of service, with unmet needs being highlighted and categorized. In considering these issues it is then necessary to outline how input from an orthogeriatric liaison team will improve patient outcomes and service delivery.

A good example of this is the scheduling of hip fracture surgery. The presence of the orthogeriatric liaison team will enable high-risk patients to be identified in advance, ensuring that the appropriate preoperative investigations are undertaken and that the patient is optimised medically, in these situations consultation with anaesthetic colleagues will also ensure that those patients with poor physical states and high operative risks are managed by senior anaesthetists and surgeons. Unnecessary delays to surgery should also be minimized, thus resulting in better patient outcomes. As previously discussed, the reduction in delays to surgery is of paramount importance if mortality rates are to be reduced. Other advantages associated with good orthogeriatric liaison will become apparent as the chapter progresses.

The scope of the service and the patient group must also be established. Will all elderly patients admitted be reviewed by the orthogeriatric liaison team or will the focus be primarily on those patients who have sustained a femoral neck fracture? Data on previous admissions need to be examined to identify the numbers and types of patients to be managed. These data will also help in the decision regarding the most appropriate model of service delivery to be utilized.

At any one time within the trauma unit at the author's university teaching hospital, there are around 55 elderly trauma patients on three wards. The mean age of these patients is 83 years. The majority have sustained a hip fracture on a background of medical, physical and/or functional frailty. In giving consideration to these factors, the criteria for review of patients by the elderly care team was established as follows:

- all patients aged over 80 years.
- all patients who had sustained a femoral neck fracture.
- patients under 80 years who had complex discharge planning needs and required intermediate care or transfer to a rehabilitation facility.

Any referral criteria must be strictly adhered to, in order to prevent the service being overwhelmed. Inappropriate referrals will affect the efficiency of service delivery to those patients who meet the inclusion criteria.

Baseline measurements for future comparison must be established. There is a plethora of reports relating to the care of the patient with a femoral neck fracture, so this information is easily obtainable and can be incorporated into the development of tools necessary for future audit. Key measurement are the length of time spent in the accident and emergency department, times to surgery, length of stay and discharge destination. Other factors that should be included are reasons for delay to surgery, readmission and mortality rates. The audit tool developed by the orthogeriatric liaison nursing team also includes data relating to time of first review by an elderly-care physician, falls investigation and secondary osteoporosis management.

Box 8.1 Osteoporosis investigation and management

Previous low-trauma fracture	Y/N	Details

Risk factors

Relevant drug history	Menopause < 50 years
Smoker	Family history
Alcohol	History of thyroid disease
Diet	Other

PSA/ESR/Bone Profile

Dexascan

Bisphosphonate/Calcichew D3 Forte/other

Members of the orthogeriatric liaison team

As well as agreeing the service needs and model, the practicalities of delivering the service and membership of the team must also be considered. In our model, the initial team members were:

- an elderly-care consultant physician with three fixed sessions per week
- an elderly-care specialist registrar seconded for 10 weeks on a rotational basis for 5 sessions per week
- a full-time older person's specialist nurse.

At this stage it is worth considering the role of the older person's specialist nurse, as there has been considerable debate about the role of specialist nurses in general and the contribution that they make to patient care. Do they, for example, enhance or de-skill the generalist nurse? What is the nature of specialist practice, and what does it mean to be a specialist practitioner? (Marshall and Luffingham 1998).

The Royal College of Nursing offers a programme leading to the award of 'Gerontological Nurse Specialist', and McCormack (1999) has clearly identified the key skills of the gerontological nurse specialist as:

> being able to demonstrate knowledge and skills of working with older people from a variety of perspectives, thereby enabling an holistic approach to understanding the needs of older people and approaches to patient care . . . in other words, an 'expert practitioner in gerontological nursing'.

A statement provided by a joint working party of the Royal College of Nursing and the British Geriatric Society outlined the benefits to individuals and services of the older person's specialist nurse and provides authoritative backing for such posts (BGS/RCN 2001).

Strong leadership skills are also a vital part of the role of the older person's specialist nurse. Several writers have cited effective nursing leadership as a major factor that will improve patient care (Cook 1999, Allen 2000). The Department of Health has also endorsed the need for effective clinical leadership (DH 1999). There has been a great deal of investment in the NHS to significantly improve nursing leadership, and the overarching aim of the Royal College of Nursing clinical leadership programme is to assist clinical leaders to develop practical strategies to improve the care that patients receive (RCN 1999).

Strong leadership skills are of particular importance when the older person's specialist nurse is working in a non-specialist elderly-care environment. In working towards rooting out age discrimination and promoting person-centred care, there will be the need to act as an excellent role model, inspiring a shared vision and demonstrating the ability to challenge the process in order to meet these goals. The older person's specialist nurses must believe in their ability to achieve results for themselves but must also have the leadership skills necessary to enable others to achieve the same end. This, as Sashkin and Rosenbach (1993) have argued, is the real job of the leader.

The older person's specialist nurse is provided with many opportunities to influence and shape the development of services and clinical practice within an acute trauma setting, and the role was considered to be pivotal in the provision of an orthogeriatric liaison service in our particular trust. Specific aims of the role were identified as follows:

- to work with older people admitted to the unit, assessing their needs and targeting interventions such as specific areas of nursing care
- to work closely with junior medical staff, nursing colleagues, allied health care professionals and social workers ensuring that person-centred care is delivered
- to liaise with elderly-care physicians and other specialists
- to challenge ageist assumptions in care and ensure that older people have access to the range of hospital services available on the same basis as other patients
- to develop practice, providing expert skills and knowledge and support to all members of the multidisciplinary team
- to work with patients, relatives and carers providing them with opportunities to express their opinions, exercise freedom of choice and feel that they are being listened to
- to ensure that patients are fully involved in decisions regarding their future rehabilitation and discharge needs.

The nursing establishment of the orthogeriatric liaison team has recently been increased, with the appointment of a full-time sister to support the nurse specialist. Another innovation has been the introduction of a secondment opportunity for junior staff nurses. The secondment is for 2 days a week and 4 months' duration, and the aim is to encourage as many junior nurses as possible to take advantage of this opportunity to enhance their knowledge of caring for older people and improve their clinical practice skills.

In providing opportunities such as these it is important to ensure that the competency of the team is developed in order to provide effective service delivery. Competency frameworks have been developed for both of the posts described above, based on the work developed by Benner and colleagues (1984, 1996) Staff nurses on secondment are exposed to all areas of service delivery under the close supervision of the nurse specialist. They are also encouraged to undertake an in-depth study of a critical incident that has occurred during the secondment and a small audit project of their choice that they then present to nursing colleagues. So far, the secondment has been positively evaluated, with one of the staff nurses having embarked on a master's-level programme of study in gerontological nursing as a result of her secondment.

Succession planning is also a key element in the delivery of the service. As with any organization, in order to develop and maintain strong leadership, it is essential that people are developed to take over senior posts (Butler and Roche-Tarny 2002).

In developing the elderly-care sister, it is important to address all the skills and competencies required to undertake the role of the nurse specialist. Regular meetings with the nurse specialist enable benchmarking of current skills against those that are actually needed. These can then be measured against the competency framework and progress can be evaluated as the elderly-care sister moves towards meeting the skills required to perform as an expert practitioner.

Within the medical team, a second consultant has also been appointed. This has provided an overall increase in current sessional consultant commitment between two consultants, reducing an individual's workload in the area of orthogeriatrics but also enabling the support of other struggling areas such as intermediate care.

Service activities and impact on patient care

Having identified the key members of the team, it is now important to explore the service activities that they undertake and the impact that these services can have on patient care. All new patients who meet the referral criteria undergo a comprehensive assessment by a member of the orthogeriatric liaison nursing team. This initial assessment, which has been explored in greater detail in earlier chapters, includes an investigation into the cause of the fall, medication review and consideration of secondary management of osteoporosis, cognitive review and social circumstances of the patient. Patients are also given the opportunity to explore their discharge plans. It is important to ensure that extreme care is taken not to replicate assessment undertaken by ward nursing staff, but to build upon that assessment and use gerontological nursing skills to synthesize the information that has been gained in order to meet specific needs of individual patients.

Pain management, deep-vein thrombosis prophylaxis, nutritional needs and fluid input and output are also reviewed in consultation with ward nursing and medical staff, with reference to the management of these specific factors in accordance to agreed protocols and practice guidelines and in relation to the needs of individual patients. Acutely ill patients or those giving cause for concern are also reviewed by the orthogeriatric liaison nursing team, with support and advice being given as required.

In responding to the needs of older people admitted to the trauma unit, it is also necessary to explore ways of working that will enhance the delivery of certain aspects of care in a more timely manner. Some patients admitted to the trauma unit have difficulties with swallowing. With limited funding for this service on the trauma directorate, response times after referral to the speech and language department could often be up to 48 hours. Patients, many of whom were undernourished prior to admission, were kept nil by mouth until a dysphagia assessment was undertaken. This obviously had implications in terms of maintaining their nutritional needs. As a result of concerns raised about this, after a period of training the older person's specialist nurse is now able to undertake dysphagia assessments. Response times following referrals have improved, with patients being seen on the day of referral, assessments undertaken and a management plan provided. On occasions, after initial assessment and when swallowing problems are extremely complex, a referral is made to a speech and language therapist. This has contributed significantly to improvements in patient care.

The presence of the elderly-care specialist registrar ensures prompt review of all new and acutely unwell patients on a daily basis. This ensures the early identification and treatment of complications, thus preventing acute deterioration which may lead to delays to surgery or even death (BOA 2003). Of key importance for the patient with a hip fracture is the high level of continuity that this service model provides, with access to an elderly-care physician on a daily basis. The elderly-care physician also alerts 'on-call' colleagues to those patients who they may be asked to review during the evening or night and at weekends. Junior and senior house officers also benefit from the support that they are given when dealing with patients who present with complex medical needs.

This support also extends to the management of patients who, because of advanced dementia, for example, present medical and nursing staff with specific ethical and legal dilemmas such as those concerning consent and nutrition. It has long been recognized that weight loss and anorexia are common in patients with advanced dementia, and the role of tube feeding in such patients continues to be controversial (Gillick 2000). The most common reason for the introduction of tube feeding is to aim to prolong life (Mitchell et al. 2000), but evidence suggests that mortality is only slightly reduced when feeding tubes are used for this group of patients (Rudberg et al. 2000). Even after feeding tubes are inserted in patients with advanced dementia there may be no improvement in nutritional status, because of the presence of cachexia-inducing cytokines (Yeh and Schuster 1999). It must also be recognized that patients with dementia do not find feeding tubes easy to tolerate.

Despite the evidence that questions the value of tube feeding in patients with dementia, it is nevertheless important to ensure that each individual case is considered on its merits and that General Medical Council and British Medical Association good practice guidelines in decision-making on withholding and withdrawing life-prolonging treatment are adhered to (BMA 2001, GMC 2002).

The orthogeriatric liaison team is in a position to provide advice and strong leadership ensuring that guidelines are adhered to and that decisions are made in a 'transparent and open manner, free from ageism and are not made in the light of resource constraints on the NHS' (BGS 2003).

Discussions with patients, carers and their families can also occur in a more timely fashion when the orthogeriatric liaison team has a daily presence on the trauma unit. The process of communication has been greatly enhanced with our own model of orthogeriatric liaison, because members of the orthogeriatric nursing team are available to discuss cases with patients, relatives and carers. The availability of the team also ensures that support is given to ward-based nursing and allied health professionals who, because of the exigencies of service delivery, may not be as easily accessible to discuss problems with patients and their carers. The elderly-care specialist registrar is also available on a daily basis to discuss problems such as acute medical deterioration of patients and the impact that this may have in relation to delays to surgery or future outcomes.

The elderly-care consultants undertake a weekly ward round on all three of the trauma wards, and are available to speak with relatives and carers when requested. The elderly-care ward round ensures regular patient review at a senior level. It also provides an excellent educational opportunity for medical, nursing and allied health professionals. Ward-based orthopaedic house and senior house officers are expected to attend the ward round, and this ensures effective communication and timely action with reference to investigation requests and referrals to other consultants and departments.

The appropriate management of femoral neck fractures is dependent upon many factors. Of key importance for the patient is the attention given to their rehabilitation and discharge planning needs. In order to meet these needs, effective communication between the various members of the multi-disciplinary team is essential. Within our model of orthogeriatric liaison it was decided to introduce weekly multi-professional team meetings on each of the trauma wards as a forum for formalizing discussions about rehabilitation and discharge planning. The introduction of the meetings was viewed by some members of the team with trepidation, with concerns over time constraints being the major issue. However, these well-coordinated meetings and the close cooperation that has been fostered between team members has done much to help improve perioperative care, rehabilitation and discharge planning. The role of multi-professional teams, rehabilitation and discharge planning is discussed in greater detail in Chapter 9.

In providing an orthogeriatric liaison service, it is important that the team are mindful of the position they are in to initiate and participate in innovative audit and research which extends beyond surgical issues. Within our own team, the older person's specialist nurse was a co-applicant on a research project funded by the NHS Research and Development Executive which examined the effectiveness and cost-effectiveness of a care pathway for femoral neck fractures (Roberts et al. 2002, Onslow et al. 2003, Roberts et al. 2004). An audit undertaken by the team also examined issues surrounding postural blood pressure monitoring. Gaps in knowledge were identified as a result of this audit, and an education programme aimed at all grades of nursing staff was introduced. Other trust policy initiatives that have been implemented, such as those relating to falls prevention and management in the acute hospital environment, are also audited regularly with the results of the audit disseminated to the individual ward managers.

Audit data relating to all aspects of care of patients with a femoral neck fracture are collected and collated by the orthogeriatric liaison nursing team. This information is disseminated regularly at audit meetings and has been influential in assisting in implementing changes in clinical practice. One illustration is the reduction in delays to surgery, which is discussed later in this chapter.

Education of staff is of key importance if a holistic approach to care is to be developed, and multi-professional teaching can do much to foster collaborative working. The orthogeriatric liaison nursing team actively participates in the unit teaching programme for nurses. An elderly-care study day for junior nursing staff is held once a year as part of their development programme. Multi-professional teaching sessions are also held on a weekly basis, with the focus not only on specific medical conditions but other salient issues including 'Essence of Care' (DH 2003a), rooting out age discrimination and breaking bad news. Supervision and education of pre-registration house officers is enhanced in the clinical environment because of the presence of the elderly-care specialist registrar who can share expert knowledge with juniors. Again; this goes beyond a focus on clinical conditions and encompasses factors such as communicating with distressed patients, relatives and carers, dilemmas in clinical decision-making and working collaboratively with other members of the multi-professional team.

The sub-role of educator has been identified in nursing literature as one of the key domains of the advanced nurse specialist/consultant nurse (Manley 1997, Ibbotson 1999, McCreadie 2001), and within our own orthogeriatric nursing liaison team this is certainly the case. Contribution to formal teaching sessions has already been alluded to, but the major educational contribution occurs at clinical level. All new members of staff and student nurses spend time with the liaison nurses and are exposed – albeit to a limited extent – to the various aspects of the role.

Dedicated time is spent working on individual wards with identified patients. In order to improve the quality of patient care it is important that we are not seen as a threat, or as judges of care delivery. Our aim is to demonstrate the efficacy of the contribution that we can make to the quality of patient care, as well as to assist nursing staff in their own professional development. By fostering collaborative working relationships with ward nursing staff we ensure that we are not seen to make all the decisions about a specific area of patient care which could prevent them from taking responsibility. It is essential that our own knowledge and skills are shared with other nursing staff, enabling them to expand their knowledge and practice that ultimately improves the delivery of patient care. Acting as effective change agents is a key aspect of our role, and the difficulty of implementing change in some areas was considered a major barrier to the development of this service. This will be explored further as the chapter progresses.

Working with patients, carers and relatives is also an important aspect of the sub-role of educator. A part of the process of education is information giving, which requires a sound knowledge of topics to be discussed and a wide range of skills in order for education to be effective (Caress 2003). Effective communication skills are essential if information is to be delivered skilfully. Our communication skills are not innate but are developed as we ourselves grow and develop, and the ability to communicate effectively is subject to a number of influences that include personal histories, personality traits and the social roles that contribute to our everyday existence. Patients will also have been subject to similar influences that will have a bearing on their communication skills. In communicating with older people it is important to be aware of these influences and the impact that 'any communication deficit might have on the individual's ability to maintain meaningful interaction with other people and the environment' (Miller 2002).

The ideal environment for giving information is one that is free from noise and distractions and affords a degree of privacy. This is often difficult in a busy ward, and the difficulty may be compounded by the factors identified above. Lack of privacy may cause patients to be more guarded when discussing the information that is shared with them. In recognition of these difficulties a dedicated room has been made available on the unit, with the older person's nurse specialist having responsibility for the booking and use of this room.

Nursing staff also need to be mindful of the timing of the information that is being given. Patients admitted with a hip fracture are likely to have some questions at or near the time of admission, but will also be shocked, distressed and even confused at this time. This may not be the best time to give too much information, and it has been our experience that limiting the amount of information at any one time and gradually building upon it helps with giving information more effectively.

Giving information verbally is beneficial for patients, but may be impeded by limited recall. For this reason we have developed supplementary written information to give to patients. It is important to note that written information should not used as a substitute for verbal information, because it is a mistake to assume that all patients will understand it (Beaver and Luker 1997). Indeed, numerous studies have highlighted the poor quality of written information that is given to patients (Petterson 1994, Scriven and Tucker 1997). Nicklin (2002) has argued that there is sufficient evidence to influence a change in practice, and has developed a protocol adapted from the work of Paley (1995) for the provision of written information, which should be extremely helpful to those charged with the writing of printed information for patients.

As well as ensuring that appropriate information is given to patients in a timely manner, taking into account the factors mentioned above, the orthogeriatric nursing team also have specialist skills in the assessment of patients. Particular attention is given to obtaining an accurate falls history, consideration of bone protection and a comprehensive social assessment. The liaison nurses are able to synthesize the information they have gained and share it with professional colleagues, ensuring that appropriate investigations and treatment are instigated. In gaining a comprehensive picture of a patients' social background, previous functional status and expressed wishes regarding their future, the orthogeriatric liaison nurses are able to ensure that appropriate and timely rehabilitation and discharge plans are made. It can be argued that these skills should be inherent in all nurses, but in developing this service the team's experience has been that this is an area of care in which we have made a significant impact, with evidence of improved rehabilitation and discharge planning that puts the patient at the centre of any care planning decisions. This is because of the advanced skills of the liaison nurses, their ability to synthesize information gained and share it with their professional colleagues. All members of the multi-professional team have also embraced the opportunities to improve their knowledge through informal and formal educational opportunities provided by the liaison nurses.

Barriers to developing and maintaining a service

Throughout this chapter the emphasis has been on the development of one particular model of orthogeriatric liaison, which, I hope, has conveyed its many good features to the reader. However, it is important to recognize that establishing and maintaining a service such as this is not without its pitfalls, and the remainder of this chapter focuses on some of these in relation to our own experiences.

At the beginning of the chapter various models of orthogeriatric liaison were introduced, with the importance of identifying the scope of the service, the patient group and resources available being highlighted as key factors in identifying the model to be followed.

Our service was originally established in 1997 with the input of one elderly-care consultant session per week to review an 18-bed fractured neck of femur ward. The ward had strict admission criteria and was aimed at those patients who had significant co-morbidities requiring intensive input from the elderly-care team. Again, as with our current model, this one had many good features and key outcome measures demonstrated the efficacy of the service with reductions in length of stay and mortality rates.

However, there were resource implications that on reflection had not been clearly identified at the developmental stage of the model. There was limited financial investment in the ward, and the nursing resources required to meet the needs of this group of patients was extremely high. The nurse/patient ratio was 1.3 nurses per bed, as opposed to 1 per bed on the other trauma wards. The number of physiotherapists or occupational therapists allocated to the ward had not been increased, despite the change in the model of service delivery on the ward. Recruitment of nursing and allied health professionals was difficult throughout the unit at this time, and there were difficulties in meeting our affordable manpower levels.

Another significant factor was that only those patients on the fractured neck of femur ward received routine, regular input from the elderly-care consultant and specialist registrar. Patients on the other wards received support from the elderly-care medical team on a consultative basis only. This was significant not only in terms of perioperative management but also with reference to the investigation and management of falls, secondary osteoporosis management and access to expert gerontological nurses. It may be argued that this resulted in an inequitable level of service provision to elderly hip fracture patients on the unit. Many lessons were learned from this experience, and the concerns highlighted – coupled with the need for one ward to be closed for several weeks because of acute nursing shortages – acted as a catalyst for seeking a new model of service delivery and led to the introduction and development of our current model.

Establishing the scope of the service, and ensuring that all members of nursing, medicine and allied health professionals are aware of it, presents another potential difficulty. In our situation consultant orthopaedic surgeons and elderly-care physicians shared responsibility for establishing procedures, protocols, communication and liaison mechanisms, but introducing new ways of delivering patient care was often fraught with difficulties. The development and implementation of an integrated care pathway (ICP) for fractured neck of femur serves as a good example of this. Development of the ICP took many months. It was difficult to get all the necessary people to the planning sessions, and it was obvious that the level of commitment from some team members was extremely poor. Some meetings took several weeks to arrange, and when they did happen, agreement on guidelines or protocols to be used was not always a foregone conclusion despite actions and timings being derived from research evidence. Despite apparent commitment to the concept of an ICP, following an extensive training programme it was obvious that ownership was not taken on by all users and its implementation was not supported at all levels (Onslow et al. 2003).

Over-reliance on the orthogeriatric liaison team was another difficulty encountered in the development of the service. Reliance on the expertise of others runs the risk of de-skilling those staff who are asking for assistance, and may also result in some staff members abdicating their responsibility. This can occur in even the most fundamental aspects of patient care: for example, a patient might be referred to the orthogeriatric liaison team because of acute confusion. In these situations, review by the elderly-care physician might reveal that even the most basic investigations such as septic screening had not been initiated. This abdication of responsibility can result in individuals not developing their own skills and knowledge, and can also lead to fragmentation in patient care.

Despite input from the orthogeriatric liaison team, difficulties were identified with regard to delays to surgery for patients with femoral neck fractures. Fewer than 50% of patients were getting to theatre within 48 hours of injury, and further analysis identified the major reason for this to be linked to issues of capacity. As previously described (pp. 122–4) a 'traffic light' system was introduced and dedicated hip fracture lists have recently been implemented. Good data collection and audit are essential in order to highlight such difficulties, and in developing a service the need for support staff to undertake audit and research activities should be identified. Currently our orthogeriatric liaison nursing staff collect, collate and present data, but considering the time taken to undertake such work it is questionable whether this are a good use of nursing resources. With appropriate education and training, an audit clerk could collect data and input it to the database. The orthogeriatric liaison nurses would, however, still need to analyse the data and disseminate the results of the data collection, as clinical knowledge is necessary in order to interpret the information.

The major aim for the older person's specialist nurse was to improve the quality of nursing care provision for older patients on the trauma unit. It is important not to underestimate the magnitude of this task, and there must be a recognition that in challenging practice there is a high risk of alienating some colleagues. Strong leadership skills and a sense of self-belief, which is considered to be an important personality trait of leadership (Howell and

Avolio 1993), are necessary to encourage nursing staff not only to share a vision but to give them a sense of ownership and participation as they are encouraged to view the care of older people as a challenge and not as a burden.

Nursing staff can be resistant to change, particularly if they are entrenched in traditional models of nursing that may not contribute positively to patient care. They may be unaware that the care they are delivering is not person-centred and that their practice is ageist. Older people are often viewed as a homogeneous group, but as Ryan (1999) has pointed out, the older population represents the most diverse of the age groups with different cohort groups having 20, 30 or even 40+ years more life experience than other 'older' people. Despite this diversity, many nursing staff reinforce the negative stereotypes of older people as frail, physically inadequate and mentally incompetent. This can manifest in ritualistic practices with little attempt at individualized care: for example, incontinence pads may be used indiscriminately because of an assumption that all older people are incontinent.

Effective communication is essential to all nursing practice, but the nursing literature provides us with a fairly bleak picture of the interactions that occur between nursing staff and older people (Warner 2000, Davies 2001). The negative stereotyping that influences some nurses can result in older people being spoken to inappropriately, with staff using secondary baby talk and patronizing speech and engaging only in superficial conversation. This can be compounded by a lack of understanding of the concepts of personhood and person-centred care, which should underpin all nursing interactions. In order to have meaningful interactions with older people it is essential that nursing staff take the time to know and understand something of their social history. An example of this is the fear experienced by a patient about the possibility of being admitted to a rest home. An exploration of her background revealed that this fear was not only related to her concerns about giving up her independence but was deeply rooted in her experience of being in institutional care throughout her childhood. This information was gained by a student nurse working with the older persons' nurse specialist. It would not have been obtained through engagement in superficial conversation, but through the development of a therapeutic relationship. Some nurses might argue that they only have time for superficial conversation, and that they are too busy to find the time to know and understand something of a person's social history. However, in the situation illustrated the information was gained while nursing staff were engaged in assisting the person to meet her personal hygiene needs, and was underpinned by an understanding of the concepts of personhood and person-centred care.

The older person's specialist nurse was and still is faced with challenges that involve dealing with negative stereotyping and ageist practice of which, as previously mentioned, nursing staff might not even be aware. That is why it is essential that time is dedicated to working with individual patients and nursing staff in the clinical environment, and this aspect of the role must not be allowed to be overtaken by other service demands.

On occasions the orthogeriatric liaison team have been met with more overt examples of ageism, as the following short conversation between an elderly-care specialist registrar and an orthopaedic surgeon illustrates:

> Elderly-care specialist registrar: 'Hello, I'm Dr X. I'm from elderly care.'
>
> Orthopaedic specialist registrar: 'Elderly – I don't care.'

This interaction between two senior members of the medical profession highlights more than anything the barriers that may be faced when developing an orthogeriatric liaison service while also attempting to root out age discrimination and promoting person-centred care. There is no magic formula, but in attempting to achieve these goals the strategies and skills that have been identified and used by our own team are:

- strong leadership skills
- a clear vision
- a sense of self-belief
- the ability to challenge the process
- a recognition that in challenging the process there is a risk of alienating some colleagues
- inspiring a shared vision
- promoting a sense of ownership and participating
- creating standards of excellence
- demonstrating clinical credibility
- modelling the way
- celebrating success.

Despite an uphill struggle in developing our particular model of orthogeriatric liaison, we do have much to celebrate in the field of orthogeriatrics at this large university teaching hospital. The effectiveness of the current liaison service has been demonstrated in several local audits and its worth was recognized by a District Audit in 1999 and a Commission for Health Improvements inspection in 2000.

The main reason for our achievement is not linked solely to the development of an orthogeriatric liaison service; it is that despite the barriers identified, most of the nursing, medical and allied health professionals have reached out and shared our vision of improving the care of older people admitted to the trauma unit. The improved support given to elderly trauma patients and the substantial improvement in the general knowledge base of nursing and medical staff working in the trauma unit has enabled us to effectively improve the quality of care delivered to elderly patients throughout their stay, and has ensured that patients' rehabilitation and discharge planning is person-centred.

CHAPTER NINE

Rehabilitation and discharge planning

Despite the commonality of their injury, patients who sustain a femoral neck fracture are not a homogeneous group. As with other aspects of care each person will present with quite different needs for rehabilitation and discharge planning. Some will be able to return home after their injury, others may require a period of intensive rehabilitation, and still others will require admission to a long-term care facility. In order to assist individuals to regain their independence or adjust to a new way of living it is therefore important to ensure coordinated, person-centred and effective team work.

Team working

At the heart of modernization of the NHS is the promotion of cooperation and partnership through improved communication and working practices across professional and organizational boundaries (Salmon and Jones 2001). Policy documents such as *The New NHS: modern and dependable* (DH 1997), *Clinical Governance: quality in the new NHS* (DH 1998a) and *A First Class Service: quality in the new NHS* (DH 1998b) have a shared vocabulary of collaboration. The *NHS Plan* (DH 2000a), *The Way to Go Home* (Audit Commission 2000) and the *National Service Framework for Older People* (DH 2001a) emphasize the potential of therapeutic working that enables and empowers older people. Throughout these ambitious policy initiatives there is an emphasis on the importance of team working, with the patient and the family being central to all team and therapeutic activity.

In order to provide effective rehabilitation and discharge planning for any patient with a femoral neck fracture, it is therefore important to ensure that team members involved in therapeutic activity have an understanding of the importance of team working.

Differing models of team working and roles within a team have been described in the academic literature. As we compare and contrast two of these models, it will become apparent to the reader that the question 'what is a team?' is not in itself an easy one to answer. However, it is important that medical staff, nurses and allied health professionals work together to unravel the complexity and dynamics of theoretical models of team working in order to ensure that health and social policy is translated into the delivery of effective care where the focus is on the patient.

What, then, is a team? We know that it is more than a group of individuals who work together. In our everyday working lives we have all been exposed to different 'teams' and have witnessed those that work well and those that don't. A team has been described as having a common focus that is agreed on, with clear roles, responsibilities, accountability and communication (Webster 2002). Another definition describes a team as 'A group in which the individuals have a common aim and in which the jobs and skills of each member fit with those of others' (Adair 1986 cited in McCormack 2001).

Thus, key elements of what constitutes a team according to these two definitions are having a shared aim and complementary roles. The importance of complementary roles has been emphasized in the work of Belbin (1998), who describes nine team roles necessary to ensure a balanced and effective team (Table 9.1)

Table 9.1 Nine roles in an effective team

Role	Role descriptor	Allowable weaknesses
Plant	Creative, imaginative, unorthodox, solves difficult problems	Ignores details. Too preoccupied to communicate effectively
Resource investigator	Extrovert, enthusiastic, communicative. Explores opportunities. Develops contacts	Over-optimistic. Loses interest once initial enthusiasm has passed
Coordinator	Mature, confident, a good chairperson. Clarifies goals, promotes decision-making, delegates well	Can be seen as manipulative. Delegates personal work
Shaper	Challenging, dynamic, thrives on pressure. Has the drive and courage to overcome obstacles	Can provoke others. Hurts people's feelings
Monitor evaluator	Sober, strategic and discerning. Sees all options. Judges accurately	Lacks drive and ability to inspire others. Overtly critical

Table 9.1 Nine roles in an effective team (continued)

Role	Role descriptor	Allowable weaknesses
Teamworker	Cooperative, mild, perceptive and diplomatic. Listens, builds, averts friction, calms the waters	Indecisive in crunch situations. Can be easily influenced
Implementer	Disciplined, reliable, conservative and efficient. Turns ideals into practical actions	Somewhat inflexible. Slow to respond to new possibilities
Completer	Painstaking, conscientious, anxious. Searches out errors and omissions. Delivers on time	Inclined to worry unduly. Reluctant to delegate. Can be a nit-picker
Specialist	Single-minded, self-starting, dedicated. Provides knowledge and skills in rare supply	Contributes on only a narrow front. Dwells on technicalities. Overlooks the 'big picture'

Source: Belbin RMC (1998) Team roles at work. Butterworth Heinemann, Oxford. Reproduced by permission.

Imbalances and ineffectiveness may result if these attributes are not evenly balanced throughout a team. If, for example, there are too many 'specialists' in a team, there may be a tendency to focus on technical aspects of care with the danger of the bigger problem being overlooked; too many 'teamworkers' could result in indecision in crisis situations.

Another key element of a team is having a shared aim. In working with the patient it is important that a shared aim is established with the patient, carers and families in order to set rehabilitation goals and plan for discharge. In the caring relationship, the partnership with the greatest potential is with patients for whom nurses (and other professionals) care (Kenny 2002). Keeping the patient at the heart of our team work seems to be an obvious factor when planning rehabilitation and discharge; however, as an illustration given later in this chapter will demonstrate, problems emerge when a common aim is not shared between professionals and patients.

When developing a team approach to patient care it is important that professionals have an understanding of different models of multi-professional team working if they are going to make the transition from working as individual practitioners towards sharing common values and beliefs and a commitment to working as part of a team.

Multidisciplinary working

The multidisciplinary model is the one most often cited in the literature as a process of team working. In this model the efforts of each member of the team are combined. There are clear boundaries between disciplines with each member of the team working towards discipline-specific goals. Thus, as Webster (2002) has suggested, such a model can be seen as reflective of uniprofessional working with the potential for professionals to work in isolation from each other but contributing to the overall treatment of the patient.

Clearly, in this model there is a need for effective communication between the various professional groups and it is important to ensure that one member of the team takes overall responsibility for the coordination of the patient's care plan, rehabilitation and subsequent discharge. Effective leadership, management and coordination is therefore key to ensuring that person-centred care occurs. However, there are inherent difficulties with this model, the most important of which is the danger of communication breakdown particularly if there is limited understanding of the roles and function of other members of the team.

In accessing the skills and expertise of the multidisciplinary team it is important for the patient to be reassured that team members are working effectively and in collaboration to meet their individual needs. Poor coordination of the team can be disastrous in terms of patient care, with the patient feeling powerless as a result of care that is uncoordinated, fragmented and poorly planned. Imagine the frustration for patients who are told by a nurse that they can be discharged as planned later that day, only to be informed by an occupational therapist a little while later that equipment is not available and therefore their discharge will not actually occur. This is a scenario that often occurs in this particular model of working, with its potential for communication breakdown, despite members of the multidisciplinary team sharing a commitment to person-centred care and collaborative working.

Professionals themselves may also become frustrated with this model of team working because of a framework of practice which involves working within the confines of professional and organizational boundaries. The clearly defined roles that they have within a team can also result in limited communication, with a multidisciplinary team meeting taking place perhaps only once a week and limited opportunity for liaison and discussion with other team members outside this defined meeting time. Changes in team membership may also occur because of, for example, occupational therapists, physiotherapists and junior medical staff rotating through different clinical areas. This can make effective team working difficult.

However, in areas where this model of team working is employed, communication barriers can be broken down if there is strong leadership and members of the team are creative in their working practices. On one trauma ward in the author's trust a rehabilitation and discharge planning communication board is used. To maintain patient confidentiality this board is kept in a non-clinical area, but is easily accessible to all members of the multidisciplinary team. The board is updated by each member of the multidisciplinary team according to interventions they have been involved in with individual patients. The communication board is also used as a focal point for multidisciplinary patient handovers. This has proved to an extremely successful method of ensuring that all members of the multidisciplinary team are kept fully engaged and updated with reference to individual patient's rehabilitation progress and discharge plans.

Interdisciplinary working

Interdisciplinary team working involves practitioners making a commitment to work with each other across professional boundaries for the benefit of the patient or client (Freeman et al. 2000). It is this model that appears to reflect most closely policies that advocate interprofessional working as a means of achieving the new agenda in the NHS, with an emphasis on the willingness of practitioners to share 'exclusive' knowledge and authority if client needs can be 'better' met by other professionals. Thus, there is a holistic approach to care with a blurring of the boundaries of professional practice.

In order to work as an interdisciplinary team there is a need to trust the judgment of other professionals, work collaboratively and demonstrate a willingness to reflect upon and change not only individual practices but also traditional ways of working with a focus on the achievement of patient-centred goals. There is much to applaud in this model which, in comparison to multidisciplinary working, does appear to take a more patient-centred approach to care, rehabilitation and discharge planning. The success of this model depends on all professionals within the team valuing true collaboration, which in turn has the potential to remove hierarchies and erode traditional power bases derived from role or function.

However, one of the main barriers to effective interdisciplinary working is a lack of encouragement or support for professional development and collaboration which may result in a lack of recognition of the potential of interdisciplinary teamwork and unwillingness by some members of the team to consider diversification of their roles. At an organizational level, there may be difficulties in striving towards the blurring of professional boundaries because of procedures and policies that professionals have to adhere to in their daily working practice. Within this framework of organizational rigidity the opportunity for effective interdisciplinary teamwork may be diminished (Barr 2000).

Both of these models of team working do share a common focus of ensuring that the patient is at the centre of team and therapeutic activity. However, with the multidisciplinary model this objective is more difficult to achieve because of the above-mentioned difficulties relating to communication. With the interdisciplinary model, the team can be seen as working much more as a whole.

Team building

Whatever model of team working is used, the importance of team building cannot be overemphasized. The development of the team is central to the delivery of effective care, and it is clear that team building needs to be based on more than a one-off team-building exercise. Team building needs to be fully integrated into daily teamwork, with an emphasis on the development of shared aims and collaborative working. Continuous and integrated team building will include:

- clinical supervision
- mentorship
- regular team meetings
- case review
- individual development plans
- reflective dialogue
- ongoing value clarification
- conflict management
- critical evaluation (McCormack 2001).

The development of the team does not depend only on team members themselves; it also needs to be recognized by managers and educationalists. Efforts are now being made within education to assist us all to develop a greater understanding of each other's roles and responsibilities and have greater skills to enhance our own professional practice. The Department of Health has recently provided funding to four pilot sites to take forward common learning in health and social care professional education. The lead programme is the New Generation Project (*www.mhbs. soton.ac.uk/newgeneration*), which is a collaboration between the Universities of Southampton and Portsmouth, and the Hampshire and Isle of Wight Workforce Development Confederation. In this initiative a radical review of the curricula has been undertaken and an integrated and interprofessional learning programme has been developed across 10 professional programmes from medicine to midwifery to physiotherapy and social work. The first cohort of 1500 students began the programme in October 2003. It is hoped that initiatives such as this will do much to improve our understanding of roles of the various professionals within a team, learning to acknowledge that all participants bring equally valid knowledge and expertise from their professional and personal experience. (Davies 2000).

Rehabilitation and discharge planning

In our exploration of teams and team working it has been clearly identified that whatever model of team working is employed, coordinated, person-centred and effective teamwork is essential in order to assist individuals to regain their independence or adjust to new ways of living. Having shared aims and complementary roles within a team are essential underpinning themes when considering rehabilitation and discharge planning for the patient with a femoral neck fracture.

Rehabilitation has been described as being concerned with lessening the impact of disabling conditions and improving the quality of life of the people with chronic illnesses particularly common among older people (Young 1996). This represents a departure from narrow definitions of rehabilitation, which tended to focus on time-limited programmes, but makes an assumption that rehabilitation always results in optimal recovery (Edwards 2002). As suggested in the opening paragraph of this chapter, this is not always the case, with some patients who sustain a femoral neck fracture making only a limited or slow recovery or not recovering at all. Thus, the emphasis of rehabilitation needs to be placed on adaptation and not just on recovery (Easton 1999) and a holistic approach should also include a concern with social, psychological and emotional health (Clay and Wade 2003).

The Audit Commission Rehabilitation Recovery Group (2000) provides us with a realistic classification of patients undergoing rehabilitation (Box 9.1).

Box 9.1 Classification of patients undergoing rehabilitation
- those who will recover quickly and do not need more than a limited amount of help with rehabilitation
- those who will take much more time and will need a lot more help
- those whose recovery will be limited and who need palliative or continuing care

Source: Audit Commission (2000). Reproduced with kind permission of HMSO.

However, it has been suggested that with the range of outcomes that might follow rehabilitation an even wider definition is called for, which not only emphasizes the promotion of optimal recovery, but also of maximizing quality of life and highlighting the importance of preventive rehabilitation that underpins all rehabilitation programmes in terms of secondary prevention, health promotion and education (Edwards 2002). Preventive rehabilitation, particularly in terms of secondary prevention, is vital in the care of patients who have sustained a femoral neck fracture. Although mobilization programmes can assist in the promotion of optimal recovery, the quality of life will be greatly enhanced if, for example, the patient is helped to overcome their fear of falling. Not all patients will make a full recovery after their injury, and in these situations the emphasis on the preventative aspect of rehabilitation also enables health professionals to recognize the importance of skills that they use to assist in the prevention of complications such as pressure sores and depression.

Another important aspect to be considered in caring for the patient with a femoral neck fracture relates to people who have cognitive impairment. Evidence suggests that patients with dementia are viewed negatively by nurses and other health professionals (Dewing 1999, Normann et al. 1999, Stokes 2000). These negative views can lead to assumptions about older people with dementia, which may result in them being denied rehabilitation opportunities because along with the label of dementia goes an accompanying belief that there is little or no potential for rehabilitation (Hancock 2003). It has to be acknowledged that there is a considerable body of evidence associating dementia with less favourable outcomes after hip fracture, with the severity of cognitive impairment being related to higher mortality and less successful return to independent living (Parker and Palmer 1995, Liebermann et al. 1996, Lyons 1997). However, in one study it was found that selected cognitively impaired patients with hip fracture were as likely as mentally normal patients to return to the community in a specialized geriatric inpatient rehabilitation programme (Goldstein et al. 1997), and a more recent study has demonstrated that geriatric assessment and intensive rehabilitation after hip fracture in patients with mild to moderate dementia diminishes the length of stay and results in significantly fewer patients being admitted to institutional care (Tiiana et al. 2000).

The rehabilitation potential for patients who have a femoral neck fracture and have a degree of cognitive impairment should not therefore be dismissed, and in this group of patients rehabilitation should not just focus on achieving functional independence. There must also be an allowance for the potential that the patient can improve cognitively, because cognition can improve over time and from place to place (Bender 2003). As Dewing has suggested it should not 'be assumed that having dementia means a complete loss of abilities, as some abilities are enhanced and new ones can be acquired' (Dewing 2003). Moreover, healthcare professionals should strive to challenge assumptions that may result in an older person with dementia being denied the same rehabilitation opportunities as other older people.

In planning rehabilitation for the older person with a hip fracture it is therefore important to recognize that rehabilitation embraces the whole person – social, emotional, physical and psychological. Rehabilitation should go beyond ensuring that a person can undertake the activities that are needed to exist, and must encompass strategies that enable people to live their life to the full.

Consideration must also be given to the environment in which rehabilitation takes place. Is an acute trauma ward the best place for rehabilitation after fixation of a hip fracture? It is usually an extremely busy and noisy environment, and often a lack of facilities for activities of daily living can result in individual patients building up a significant deficit of activity in their own progression because of the acute nature of the ward environment. If rehabilitation does not take place on an acute trauma ward, what are the alternatives and do they offer better outcomes for the patients?

Evidence suggests that older people who are admitted to hospital stay there longer than younger people (Stevenson and Spencer 2002). This is often due to a social and psychological process known as institutionalization, and the quite rapid loss of life skills and social function that can occur when an older person is looked after in a typical acute ward environment. These problems have been highlighted in a report from the Royal Commission on long term care (Sutherland 1999).

Over the last decade rehabilitation services for older people have received a great deal of attention from policy-makers. Concerns with demographic trends, an increasing awareness of the need to use scarce resources cost-effectively, recognition of the pivotal role of rehabilitation in elderly care, the objective of reducing acute hospital lengths of stay and cost-containment initiatives represent some of the factors that have resulted in rehabilitation of older people acquiring an increasingly important profile for both policy-makers and service providers within health and social care agencies (Ward et al. 2004). The impetus of the intermediate care agenda which, according to the Department of Health would 'provide a range of integrated services to promote faster recovery from illness, prevent unnecessary acute hospital admission, support timely discharge and maximize independent living' (DH 2002c), has also contributed to the interest in seeking alternative care environments for the rehabilitation of older people.

Rehabilitation facilities offered to hip fracture patients include intermediate care, which can include early supported discharge schemes, geriatric orthopaedic rehabilitation units and mixed geriatric rehabilitation units. Evidence in relation to each of these has been reviewed by the NHS Research and Development Health Technology Assessment Programme (Cameron et al. 2000). This review suggests that early supported discharge schemes are only suitable for a subset of less disabled patients, that they are cost-effective, shorten length of stay and increase rates of return to previous residential status. Other studies point to the psychological benefits to patients with early supported discharge schemes (Sander 2002, Cunliffe et al. 2004). There is no evidence that length of stay in a geriatric orthopaedic rehabilitation unit is less than in a conventional orthopaedic unit or a mixed geriatric rehabilitation unit, suggesting that geriatric orthopaedic rehabilitation units are unlikely to be cost-effective. However, some frail older people may benefit, with reduced rates of re-admission or need for admission to nursing homes (Health Help the Aged 2000). A recent Cochrane Review concluded that although a number of studies have investigated rehabilitation environments and identified factors that may impact on rehabilitation outcomes, the lack of rigorous research design makes it difficult to draw conclusions about the various rehabilitation environments (Ward et al. 2004).

Whatever the environment, it is important that professionals working with patients to meet their rehabilitation needs recognize that many older people fear dependency and value being able to undertake normal activities (Bowling and Grundy 1997). As previously noted, various professional groups contribute to the rehabilitation of older people and all of their contributions should be recognized. It is acknowledged that, because they are there all day and all week during a patient's stay in hospital (or other rehabilitation facilities), nurses provide continuity in the rehabilitation process (Law 2003). However, many nurses have difficulty in articulating their role in rehabilitation and it is often not recognized or valued by nurses themselves (Luker and Waters 1996). In seeking to clarify the role of nurses in rehabilitation nursing, the Royal College of Nursing has identified eight categories relating to the role (Figure 9.1). These eight categories act as a framework which can assist nurses to articulate the extent of their contribution to the rehabilitation process.

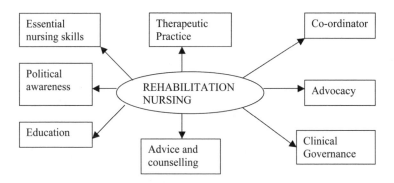

Figure 9.1 Categories in rehabilitation nursing (Royal College of Nursing 2000).

Discharge planning

Early assessment by medical, nursing and allied health professionals to formulate appropriate preliminary rehabilitation plans has been shown to facilitate rehabilitation and discharge (Audit Commission 1995, 2000) of patients who have sustained a femoral neck fracture, with premorbid mental state, function and mobility being the most reliable predictors of the success of rehabilitation (Audit Commission 1995, 2000). It is recommended that within 48 hours of admission a corroborated history should be obtained, which should include:

• premorbid function and mobility
• available social support
• current relevant clinical conditions
• mental state (SIGN 2002).

If these are not fully assessed on admission, there may be delays to discharge. Postoperative rehabilitation plans may be unrealistic if there is a lack of information about a person's previous function, and if social circumstances are not fully assessed on admission there may be delays in addressing problems once a patient is fit and ready for discharge.

As with any assessment, it is important that the assessor builds a trusting relationship with the patient. Without a sense of trust and a feeling of being listened to in a calm and unhurried manner, patients will have difficulty in sharing personal information and may be reluctant to discuss vulnerabilities that they might have. Spending time with patients and using good interpersonal skills are therefore key to building relationships (Keady and Bender 1998).

It has been suggested that in older people previous mobility is often more important than diagnosis in predicting outcomes (Goldstein et al. 1997, Heruti et al. 1999) Assessment of previous mobility provides a baseline against which realistic goals can be set and progress measured. Information to be obtained is listed in Box 9.2.

Box 9.2. Assessment of previous mobility
• Do the patients usually mobilize with or without a mobility aid? The type of mobility aid needs to be identified, e.g. stick, frame, electric scooter. Other modes of assisted mobilization must also be considered, e.g. furniture walking.
• Do the patients usually go outside, and if so do they go out by themselves or do they need assistance?
• Are the patients able to climb stairs and if not, what are the limiting factors?

- Are the patients car drivers?
- Are there any other factors that impact on their mobility, e.g. unstable gait, fear of falling, chronic pain, cognitive impairment?
- Roughly how far could they walk before they sustained their hip fracture?

It is important to explore with patients how they believe they are coping in terms of their mobility, whether they have experienced any deterioration in their mobility over recent months and how they anticipate they will manage in the future. Corroborative information from a family member or caregiver is also important. This needs to be done sensitively, recognizing that there may be a difference in perception about how people were mobilizing before admission to hospital. Obtaining corroborative information from a family member or caregiver raises important questions: for example, would corroborative information be sought when considering the rehabilitation needs of a younger person? In attempting to answer this question it must be recognized that such information will only be sought in circumstances where professionals might have concerns about future rehabilitation and discharge planning. For instance, if we consider people living alone at home who have had previous falls and use a Zimmer frame to aid mobility, those individuals may believe that they are coping well with their mobility but family members might raise concerns that the patients are not actually using their mobility aids and this has contributed to their frequent falls. Information such as this would be vital in working with the individual to plan future rehabilitation goals. Thus, as with other aspects of patient care, considerations relating to the obtaining corroborative information must be based on a high standard of initial assessment and, wherever possible, consent should be obtained from the patient before seeking this information.

Functional ability

In assessing previous functional ability it is necessary to consider how individuals carry out activities that most people take for granted. How, for example, do they manage to use the toilet, wash and dress? A validated assessment tool such as the Barthel Activities of Daily Living Score (Mahoney and Barthel 1965) can be used as an index for recording what patients are usually able to do. When considering rehabilitation and discharge planning this index can then be used with patients to set realistic goals for the future. Again, it is important to seek corroborative information when at all possible, as many older people have a fear of losing their independence and may not wish to acknowledge that they have been finding it increasingly difficult to do things that they previously took for granted.

Mental state

Assessment of cognitive function is discussed at length in Chapter 5. For the purpose of discharge planning, it is essential that careful assessment is undertaken so that the right care can be provided. An understanding of the patient's previous lifestyle and past history is important; someone who has recently developed confusion requires very different care from an elderly person who has long-term memory loss. Early and full involvement of the patient's relatives and/or carers is also important.

Social circumstances

It is clearly important to gain a picture of patients' social circumstances. The condition of patients' homes and how they are able to function in that environment needs to be identified in order to work with them in establishing realistic rehabilitation goals and good discharge planning. The patients may, for example, have stairs to climb and only have upstairs toilet facilities, so a realistic goal would be to ensure that patients are able to go up and down stairs safely before discharge. However, circumstances might dictate that they can no longer able to manage stairs as a result of their hip fracture, and it may be necessary to negotiate alternatives. For example, patients might be able to adapt a room downstairs and willing to use a commode, if it means that they are to remain at home. Such negotiations need to be handled sensitively and it should be recognized that these changes cause enormous upheaval not only to the patients but also to other family members who may be sharing their home.

Current social support, whether informal or formal, should be discussed with patients. The individuals' preferences for the future, and the view of relatives and/or carers must also be taken into account. Again, there may be differences in perception of the situation, with the amount of informal support that is being provided needing careful consideration. Carers who provide a substantial amount of care on a regular basis are by law (The Carers [recognition and services] Act 1995) entitled, on request, to an assessment of their ability to care or continue care, and it is important to ensure that health service professionals are aware of this fact in order to support those carers who request an assessment.

If patients usually live in residential or nursing home accommodation, criteria for transfer back need to be established early, with ward staff liaising closely with residential and nursing home staff regarding patient progress and potential discharge date.

In acknowledging that discharge planning should begin on the day of admission, it is also important to recognize that it is a dynamic process that should be ongoing throughout patients' hospital stay. Different levels of discharge planning are required for different older people, and any assessment should not be influenced by the existing range of services or the financial status of the service user, but should clearly set out the needs of older people (BGS 2004).

Most older people are discharged promptly from acute NHS hospital care. However, on average an older person admitted to hospital as an emergency will stay in hospital more than 50% longer than the average length of stay for all adults (National Audit Office 2003) and a report by the Department of Health identified that in September 2002, 8.9% of older people occupying NHS acute care beds had their discharge from hospital delayed, equating to 4150 older patients on any given day (DH 2003d). For older people, a protracted length of stay brings with it inherent risks of infection, loss of independence and confidence. The important contribution made by carers can be neglected and their concerns marginalized, which can lead to unexpected difficulties later in the discharge planning process (National Audit Office 2003).

The NHS Plan (DH 2000a) identified the need for a simplification of the assessment process operating within the NHS and between the NHS and councils with social services responsibility. The single assessment process has been introduced for older people in an attempt to overcome some of the longstanding problems inherent in a system where people with complex needs often undergo multiple and uncoordinated assessments (DH 2001e).

Delays that occur in the discharge planning process are often predictable, with many of them relating to communication and coordination between health and social care and between primary and secondary care, and others relating to internal hospital systems (HCHC 2001–2). These factors underline the importance of starting discharge planning as early as possible after admission in order to plan for problems and resolve them before they impact on patient care and length of stay.

The Community Care (delayed discharges etc.) Act 2003 (DH 2003d) places duties upon the NHS and councils with social services responsibilities in England relating to communication between health and social care systems around the discharge of patients and communication with patients and carers. The NHS is required to notify councils of any patient's likely need for community care services, and their proposed discharge date. A system of reimbursement has also been introduced for delayed hospital discharges if the council has not put in place services that the patient or carers need for discharge to be safe; the council will pay the NHS a charge per day of delay. Thus, since January 2004, councils have had a financial incentive to assess people promptly and transfer them from an acute ward to a more appropriate setting as soon as they are ready for discharge.

With these incentives, and pressure on acute care beds, it is important to ensure that patients with femoral neck fracture are actually safe for discharge. Guidance from the health and social care change agent team/reimbursement implementation team sets out three criteria for making the decision emphasizing that all three criteria should be addressed at the same time whenever possible:

• a clinical decision is made that the patient is ready for transfer AND
• a multidisciplinary team decision has been made that the patient is ready for transfer AND
• the patient is safe to transfer/discharge (DH 2003c).

Premature discharge can result in poor preparation of the patient for going home, and some needs may be unmet. Assumptions may also have been made about the ability of carers to cope. Again, it is important to recognize that effective and efficient discharge practices are necessary to avoid premature discharges and prevent an increase in re-admissions to hospital (DH 2001f).

As suggested at the start of this chapter, for some patients who have sustained a femoral neck fracture a return home may not be possible. It is essential in these circumstances that the risks faced by older people at home are balanced by the risks to their health and quality of life by an unwelcome move to residential or nursing care (BGS 2004). Discharging older people from an acute hospital bed to long-term residential or nursing care is not ideal, and it is important to ensure that every effort has been made to optimize their rehabilitation potential before such a life-changing decision is considered. An opportunity of continued rehabilitation should be considered and offered whenever possible, to enable people to have longer to prepare for or consider other alternatives to long-term care. The case study below offers some insight into the difficulties experienced when a patient is faced with the difficult decision of transfer to a long-term care facility.

Case study 1

Mrs X was a 93-year-old woman who lived alone in a warden-controlled flat. She had poor mobility and had for the past two years spent her days and nights sitting and sleeping in an armchair in her lounge. She had meals delivered seven days a week and a daily visit from carers to assist with personal hygiene and for the emptying of a bucket which she used to urinate in as needed. She was able to shuffle slowly to the toilet once a day to open her bowels. Whilst attempting to stand and use her bucket to urinate into she fell and sustained a femoral neck fracture that resulted in admission to hospital. Following surgery she made a good postoperative recovery but her mobility was extremely poor and despite intensive physiotherapy she was only able to stand and transfer from bed to chair with maximum assistance from two people.

When exploring her preferences for discharge she clearly expressed a wish to go home, advising the occupational therapy staff that she had an electric bed in her bedroom and suggesting the possibility of using a hoist to assist in transfer from bed to chair. She was adamant that she would be able to stand herself to use her bucket, and at times appeared to have little insight into how her elimination needs could be managed with her limited mobility. Her niece usually visited her once a week and, while expressing concerns about her aunt's increasing frailty, she was keen to ensure that all options were explored regarding her discharge. An access visit to Mrs X's home by the occupational therapist revealed that there was in fact no room for a hoist in the flat, and the physiotherapist believed that Mrs X had reached the optimal level of mobility that she was going to achieve.

A case conference was organized and on the day of the meeting Mrs X stated that she felt like a 'prisoner going before the judge and jury'. After a great deal of discussion Mrs X agreed that it would be in her best interest to move into a rest home (she felt that she needed to do this to allow peace of mind for her niece). In discussing the outcome of the case conference with her, it was apparent to the older person's specialist nurse that Mrs X was deeply troubled about a transfer to a rest home. Over the next few days they had many conversations, with the focus for Mrs X being on the fact that she would not see her flat again 'It's just the thought of never seeing my flat again'. The older person's specialist nurse conveyed her concerns about Mrs X to other members of the multidisciplinary team and questioned whether the team had achieved all they could in attempting to transfer MrsX back to her own home. All members of the multidisciplinary team agreed that transfer home would not be a safe option for her.

After liaison with Mrs X, her niece and the social worker, arrangements were made for Mrs X to visit her flat before her transfer to the rest home. Mrs X was also reassured by the fact that she would not need to sell her flat immediately as she had adequate finances to support herself in the rest home for at least six months, and that she would be able to take treasured possessions and small items of furniture with her.

Mrs X was sad and less communicative during her final days on the acute ward as she prepared for transfer to her new rest home. She was able to visit her flat to say goodbye, and subsequent discussion with the social worker revealed that Mrs X had settled well into her new rest home and of her own volition had instructed her niece to sell her flat.

For the patient in this case study sustaining a femoral neck fracture had a devastating effect on her quality of life, resulting in a decline in ambulatory status and subsequent admission to residential care. It is questionable whether she made the move to the rest home from her own free choice or because of pressure put on her by her niece and members of the multidisciplinary team. It is worth reflecting on this case study and considering how things could have been managed differently, and, if managed differently, what would the outcome have been in terms of quality of life for this woman?

Some patients with a femoral neck fracture may never recover from their injury and it is equally important that in the discharge planning process, person-centred care is provided when a patient reaches the end stage of their life. In the second case study, it is evident that the rhetoric of person-centred care can be translated into reality when the expressed wishes of the patient and family/carers remain central to care.

Case study 2

Mrs W was a 97-year-old woman who sustained a femoral neck fracture after falling at her rest home. She had advanced dementia and had lived in the rest home for a few months, having previously shared a home with her youngest daughter and her family. The daughter and her five siblings obviously cared greatly for their mum. Mrs W's condition fluctuated a great deal after surgery, but over time it became apparent that she was not going to recover and her care needs had increased significantly. The idea of nursing home placement was discussed at a multidisciplinary team meeting and the elderly-care consultant discussed this option with the family. They asked to wait for a further week before any decision was made, in the hope that their mother might make some improvement. The older person's specialist nurse subsequently had discussions with two of the daughters when it became clear that Mrs W was not going to get better. They expressed a wish to take their mother home because they wanted her to die in familiar surroundings with the family caring for her (they had always been actively engaged in her care on the ward). They also expressed some concerns that their wishes would not be met because some staff told them that it would be better for Mrs W to stay on the ward because of her worsening condition. By this stage it was clear that Mrs W's condition was rapidly deteriorating and that she would not survive much longer. The elderly-care consultant was concerned that she might not survive the journey home, and some nursing staff shared these concerns, but although the family acknowledged these issues they were still keen to take their mother home.

Having listened to their wishes, which they suggested would have also been what their mother would have wanted, every effort was made to expedite the safe transfer of Mrs W from hospital to home. The rapid response and district nursing services were contacted, as well as the GP and local pharmacist. Mrs W was transferred home within 30 minutes of the decision being made for her transfer. A rapid response nurse and district nursing sister met the patient as she arrived home. She died peacefully in the early hours of the next morning, with her family at her bedside.

After the death of Mrs W her family expressed extreme gratitude to all the staff involved in ensuring that they were able to have their mum at home for the last few hours of her life. She was at home with them for less than 24 hours, but they were relieved that she spent those last few precious hours in her own home, surrounded by her family. The GP commented that their grieving process had been helped because they had followed their mother's wishes and that health and social care services had responded to their needs.

When reflecting on the discharge of this patient, one nurse wrote that she felt an enormous sense of satisfaction because the patient had received truly person-centred care and the rhetoric of providing seamless care had been translated into reality for this patient and her family. It was a reflection that was echoed by the family, the community nurses, the rapid response service and the GP.

Clearly, coordinated rehabilitation and discharge planning is essential to assist individuals to regain their independence or adjust to new ways of living following a femoral neck fracture, so that timely and appropriate discharge occurs with avoidable delays to discharge and re-admission to hospital being prevented. Underpinning this is an emphasis on collaborative working between all members of the multi-professional team and at the primary and secondary health and social care interface. The patient and family and/or carers must at all times be central to all team and therapeutic activity if person-centred rehabilitation and discharge planning is to be achieved.

CHAPTER TEN

Impact of policy on the care of the patient with a hip fracture

Concerns about the care of older people in acute hospital settings have become a major feature of policy and debate in the NHS in recent years. The profile of older people and their experience of acute health care delivery was considerably raised by the *Observer* newspaper and Help the Aged's 'dignity on the ward' campaign, which highlighted the appalling conditions of care that some older people experienced in acute hospitals (Help the Aged 2000). A plethora of reports by statutory and non-statutory organizations have further challenged our approach to older people in the various care settings in which they present themselves.

The purpose of this chapter is to attempt to identify the key reports and policies that are particularly relevant to the care of older people with hip fracture. In considering these, attention will be drawn not only to the impact that they have on patients and their carers but also on those professionals charged with their implementation. Several major reports related specifically to the care of the patient with a hip fracture have been produced, and these reports have been influential in assisting us to question, challenge and seek out ways of working that will help us to improve the care that is delivered to this group of patients. The following reports listed below are of particular significance, and all professionals involved in the care of hip fracture patients should have a working knowledge of them and an understanding of the recommendations that they contain:

- The East Anglian Hip Fracture Audit (Todd et al. 1995, Laxton et al. 1997)
- *United They Stand* (Audit Commission 1995, 2000)
- SIGN Guideline 56 (SIGN 2002)
- *The Care of Fragility Fracture Patients* (BOA 2003)

Several key themes have emerged from these reports:

- Patients should be assessed immediately in the Accident and Emergency Department and measures should be in place to 'fast track' patients to ward areas.
- Operations should be carried out, or supervised, by a consultant or specialist registrar.

- Operations on medically fit patients should be performed within 24 hours of admission.
- Physicians who specialize in the care of older people should be involved in the care of hip fracture patients.
- Recovery after a fracture can be improved if services are well planned and coordinated from the time patients first enter hospital until their discharge.
- Patients should be rehabilitated as soon as possible.

It has also been recognized in many of reports listed above that the care of hip fracture patients is a good indicator of the quality of acute and primary care services for older people in general. This is because patients who sustain a hip fracture have a defined starting point to their journey of care (when they sustain their injury). Many of them have complex needs and may also require a wide range of services. Thus, it could be argued that in examining the care that this group of patients receives, the information could be extrapolated and used as a means for benchmarking the quality of care delivered to all older people who use health and social care services.

The key themes that have emerged from the reports mentioned above can be regarded as a framework which can be further built upon to improve the delivery of services for older people who sustain a hip fracture. Other key priorities that have emerged in the management of patients with a hip fracture include, for example, the importance of nutrition and pain management. Indeed, some of the reports have also highlighted these salient factors when considering the overall quality of patients' experience.

Although authoritative and highly influential in the shaping of hip fracture service delivery, these reports only provide guidelines and recommendations for practice and it is up to individual NHS trusts to as do as they see fit with the recommendations and guidelines. Even when NHS trusts strive to meet these recommendations, they can fall short of the standards identified. For example, despite strenuous efforts, the 1-hour target for fast tracking in A&E departments recommended by the Royal College of Physicians (RCP 1989) has proved almost impossible to achieve (Rajmohan 2000, Dinah 2003).

According to recommendations in the reports, operations should be carried out within 24 hours of injury in medically fit patients and there is a considerable body of evidence pointing to increased mortality rates if surgery is delayed (Audit Commission 1995, 2000, SIGN 2002). However, in practice delays to surgery often occur, for many reasons. Orthopaedic surgeons working on busy trauma units are faced daily with the difficult task of prioritizing patients for surgery. Often their decisions are not only based on clinical priorities but may be affected by a number of operational factors such as lack of capacity, matching appropriately experienced anaesthetists with the complexity of the type of patient and surgical treatment, availability of theatre equipment and appropriately skilled theatre staff. Other factors such as the availability of radiography staff can also have an impact upon delays to surgery. In tertiary referral centres, orthopaedic surgeons may also be faced with difficult decisions about the acceptance of complex cases from other units, which will almost inevitably have an impact on times to surgery for the local population, some of whom may have hip fractures.

Even when key themes for good hip fracture care are used to assist in the audit of clinical practice and service delivery, they are of little benefit if NHS trusts do not act on their findings and ensure effective and efficient targeting of resources in the care of patients with hip fracture. Despite some of these apparent difficulties in the implementation of these key recommendations, it is nevertheless important to acknowledge that they can be a powerful guide in assisting us to meet our primary aim – enhancing the care of older people with hip fractures. In a large number of orthopaedic units throughout the UK there is evidence of the development of good models of orthogeriatric liaison, with efforts being made to standardize and streamline hip fracture care, using the key themes identified in these influential reports to shape and drive the delivery of services to this patient group.

Although the abovementioned reports and guidelines relate specifically to the care of hip fracture patients, there are a number of other influential publications that have an impact upon the care of older patients with hip fracture and in the following sections we consider some of these.

Essence of Care

As previously mentioned, the profile of older people and their experience of acute health care service delivery was considerably raised by the 'dignity on the ward' campaign (Help the Aged 2000). Of considerable concern to older people and their carers was the lack of dignity, respect and privacy that they were afforded during their experiences of acute hospital care. Other concerns related to shortcomings in fundamental and essential aspects of care. The NHS plan (DH 2000a) reinforced the importance of 'getting the basics right' and improving the patient's journey and experience. In February 2001 the Essence of Care (current edition DH 2003a) was launched. This arose from a commitment to improve the quality of fundamental and essential aspects of care, and has contributed to the introduction of clinical governance in organizations by ensuring that benchmarking is used to improve the quality of fundamental and essential aspects of care.

The Essence of Care uses benchmarking tools to measure the existing standard of nine areas of care (see Box 10.1), highlighting where improvements need to be made. Benchmarking can be regarded as a patient-focused good practice guide that is centred on the needs of patients and their carers. The Essence of Care can be used as a framework for assessment, the development of core care plans and the identification of measurable outcomes. It will also assist us in determining quality versus quantity when examining the care that is being delivered. Clinical practitioners are able to compare, celebrate and share good practice and ensure that plans are developed to overcome weaknesses in practice.

Box 10.1 Essence of Care: nine fundamental aspects of care

- Principles of self care
- Privacy and dignity
- Record keeping
- Food and nutrition
- Continence/bladder/bowel care
- Pressure ulcers
- Personal and oral hygiene
- Safety of patients with mental health needs
- Communication with patients/users/carers

Source: DH (2003a). Reproduced with kind permission of HMSO.

The nine benchmarks identified in the Essence of Care are extremely significant in evaluatinge the care of the patient with a hip fracture. When using Essence of Care benchmarking, it is important that changes and improvements focus on the indicators that have been identified by patients, carers and professionals because it is these items that are important in achieving the benchmarks of good practice. It is also necessary to acknowledge that all sets of benchmarks are interrelated; for example, elements of privacy and dignity link with continence and bladder and bowel care (NHS 2003a).

Clearly, the main driver for the introduction of the Essence of Care was the need to support measures to improve the quality of patient care, and any initiative such as this needs commitment not only at ward level but throughout the whole of any organization. There are therefore several important questions about the implementation of the Essence of Care. For example, do we as professionals have the right skills to undertake benchmarking, and do we have a clear understanding of the process? In order to ensure that we do, all staff must have an understanding of the philosophy underpinning the Essence of Care, and all health care personnel need to be adequately trained in the use of the toolkit. The Essence of Care also needs to be fully integrated into the educational curriculum of our future health care professionals.

We also need to question how we know whether or not we are doing things right in terms of the delivery of patient care. Is there, for example, easily accessible, evidence-based research which can assist us with and inform our practice? Is the evidence base regularly updated, and what measures are in place to disseminate this information? How do we monitor patient care? Patient narratives and observations of care are two extremely powerful tools at our disposal for measuring the quality of the service that we deliver to our patients, and as more practitioners undertake leadership programmes it is likely that these two tools will be increasingly used as a way of informing the benchmarking process. The reporting of clinical incidents, identification of environmental and clinical risks and the taking forward of these issues in terms of the dissemination of actions will also contribute significantly to the benchmarking process. Most importantly, the views of patients and their carers need to be taken into consideration and the role of patient forums and patient advocacy and liaison services are of key significance in moving things forward in terms of the Essence of Care (DH 2003a).

There is a need to ensure that there is an identified lead for each clinical team involved with Essence of Care clinical benchmarking. Accountability and responsibility arrangements need to be clear, and it is necessary to ensure that Essence of Care benchmarking is clearly integrated into any directorate business plan with a clear reporting framework to inform individual NHS trust boards of progress being made and barriers that impede that progress.

Although Essence of Care benchmarking may provide practitioners with more work in the initial stages, the results are measurable and staff quickly become familiar with the tool. The use of the benchmarking tool helps them to feel empowered to take an active part in examining their practice and take control over what they do. In moving towards best practice they can celebrate and share their success, and truly feel that they are making a difference.

The National Service Framework for Older People

National Service Frameworks are described as a way of 'setting standards that will achieve greater consistency in the availability and quality of services for a range of major care areas and disease groups. The aim is to reduce unacceptable variations in care and standards of treatment, using best evidence of clinical and cost-effectiveness' (DH 1998a). The National Service Framework for Older People was launched in 2001, following a senior-level enquiry that considered what was being done well and what needed to be improved in terms of caring for our older population (DH 2001a). A wide range of outside organizations, older people and their carers were also consulted. The National Service Framework provides us with a 10-year programme of action intended to ensure that older people have fair access to high-quality integrated health and social services. Implicit in its aims is ensuring that the needs of older people are at the heart of the reform programme for health and social care, ensuring that:

- High-quality care and treatment is provided on the basis of need regardless of age.
- Care is person-centred with services fitting around peoples' needs.
- Older people are treated as individuals, with their privacy and dignity being maintained at all times.
- There is fair distribution of resources for those conditions that most affect older people.
- Older people's health and independence is promoted.
- The financial burden of long-term care is eased.

For patients who have sustained a hip fracture, their families and carers and the professionals involved in their care the key question is how the standards identified in the National Service Framework will improve the overall experience of their acute hospital stay and beyond, and how they can ensure that these standards are being met. The need for a National Service Framework for older people was triggered by concerns about widespread infringement of dignity and unfair discrimination in older people's access to care (DH 2001a) – for example, older patients being less likely to receive appropriate treatment than younger patients with similar injuries in trauma units (Grant et al 2000). Negative staff attitudes can also have an impact on the quality of care delivered to older patients in many different care settings (HAS 1999).

Rooting out age discrimination is Standard One of the National Service Framework, with the aim of ensuring that older people are 'never unfairly discriminated against in accessing NHS or social care services as a result of their age' (DH 2001a). In terms of access to an acute trauma bed following a hip fracture, it can be argued that this standard is being met. However, in some circumstances – for example, delays to surgery in medically fit patients – de facto discrimination can and does occur, because we are aware that delaying surgery has a more detrimental effect in older people than in younger adults and yet despite this knowledge, for various operational reasons, this continues to be a key issue in many trauma units.

In order to reassure patients with a hip fracture that they are not discriminated against because of their age, it is important that they are kept fully informed and involved in decisions about their treatment and future care. Although there are clinical and practice champions within each organization to lead in the professional development of staff in caring for older people and meeting the National Service Framework standards, it is also important that clinical staff at ward level have the necessary skills and confidence in working with older people to ensure that behaviour is not perceived as discriminatory. It may be difficult to meet the standard of rooting out age discrimination if the expertise in terms of care of older people is not available, and if there is not a clear line of accountability for ensuring that this key standard is implemented. Older persons' nurse specialists are now employed on many trauma units, and this can be seen as a positive step towards ensuring that age discrimination is tackled through good leadership and management. It is also important that patients with a hip fracture receives good ongoing care on a trauma ward, which will involve several key elements identified in Standard Four of the National Service Framework and clearly link to Essence of Care clinical benchmarking: for example, nutritional status and risk management, continence risk management and pressure sore risk management.

When considering other standards in the National Service Framework in terms of the care of patients with a hip fracture, it is important to ensure that there is robust provision of service for the treatment and management of patients, who in almost all cases have sustained their hip fracture as a result of a fall. Patients need to be reassured that the cause of the fall will be fully investigated and that treatment as a result of the investigation will be provided. New specialist teams have been set up throughout the NHS to improve the treatment, care and rehabilitation of older people who are injured as a result of a fall, and a key milestone of Standard Six (falls) of the National Service Framework is that by 2005 all primary care trusts should have a fully integrated falls service. It is important that on discharge from hospital the patient is assessed and has access to a community falls service as required. Although there is a great deal of emphasis on the treatment and management of falls, it is also important for patients to receive the best possible care in terms of the treatment of osteoporosis, and patients who are admitted with hip fractures should have access to osteoporosis services and treatment according to their individual clinical needs.

As suggested in Chapter 8, it is recommended that there should be at least one ward in every acute hospital that is a centre of excellence for the care of patients with hip fracture. Whatever model of service provision is used, patients need reassurance that the care that they receive is evidence based and includes the early and continued involvement of a physician who specializes in the care of older people (Standard Four). Evidence from the Audit Commission report (2000) suggests that in some areas this is still not the case, and this is indeed worrying in terms of the co-morbidities that many patients with hip fracture present with and their ongoing need for rehabilitation.

Can we reassure patients with a hip fracture that their privacy and dignity will be maintained when they come into hospital? If we think of the concerns raised in the 'dignity on the ward' campaign and consider the distress that being in a mixed-sex ward can cause to older people, it is reassuring that government investment of £120 million has gone towards the modernization of many old 'Nightingale' wards to provide single-sex accommodation, reduce noise and improve privacy. However, because of difficulties with bed availability, older people are still sometimes admitted to mixed-sex bays. Fundamental issues of privacy and dignity can be overlooked: for example, ill-fitting curtains that do not adequately screen patients when intimate and personal care is being delivered, and the sharing of mixed-sex toilet facilities. Modern matrons and older persons' champions are in key positions to challenge these practices and work with trust boards to attempt to rectify the difficulties.

Maintaining privacy and dignity is also an integral part of the provision of person-centred care. As described in the National Service Framework, person-centred care aims to ensure that 'older people are treated as individuals and they receive appropriate and timely packages of care that meets their needs as individuals, regardless of health and social service boundaries' (Standard Two). Older people and their carers have not always been treated with respect or with dignity (HAS 1998, 2000). Using the Essence of Care toolkit can help in monitoring the quality of care, in terms of maintaining privacy and dignity and in any evaluation of care or services for older people. In order to assist patients with a hip fracture to make informed decisions about their future care they need to be provided with proper information about their own health, assessment, diagnosis, treatment, rehabilitation and care, any referral procedures or eligibility criteria. It is only with this information that they can make informed choices about their future care options and the level of risk that they are prepared to take when making these choices. Professional staff must be knowledgeable about the services available in order to provide accurate information and to assist patients and carers with the decisions that they make.

In terms of rehabilitation of patients with a hip fracture, a key element of the National Service Framework is the expansion of rehabilitation services and the provision of extra intermediate care beds. As previously identified (Chapter 8), there are several different models of orthogeriatric rehabilitation and each of these has been thoroughly reviewed by the Cochrane Collaboration (Cameron et al. 2003). It appears that intermediate care services could have a positive effect in terms of rehabilitation and discharge planning for some patients who have sustained a hip fracture, but we must question how responsive to demand these services are. There may be a danger of losing specialist geriatric rehabilitation units in order to free money for the purchasing and provision of 'extra' intermediate care services. It can be argued that a specialist geriatric rehabilitation unit is of key importance for patients who have sustained a hip fracture and require rehabilitation over a long period of time in order to make non-spontaneous recovery happen (Evans and Tallis 2001).

If patients are to be referred to community rehabilitation teams on discharge from the acute care environment, it is important that these teams are able to respond and provide services in a timely manner. We would not consider sending a patient home if the care package they required was not in place, yet in some circumstances a patient may wait several weeks after referral for review by a community rehabilitation team. There are many reasons for this, such as inappropriate referrals to the service and shortages of staff. It is important that in these circumstances patients are made aware of the delay, and in sending patients home, professionals must be certain that such delays will not be detrimental to the progress made by the patient in terms of functional recovery.

Intermediate care beds in non-acute care settings can offer the opportunity for hip fracture patients to make a rapid, but sustained transition back to their usual place of residence. Eligibility criteria for admission to an intermediate care facility must be clearly identified and agreed by all members of the multi-professional team, and in developing these criteria the focus should be kept on the key objectives of intermediate care which, in terms of the patient with a hip fracture, are to facilitate timely discharge from hospital, promote effective rehabilitation and minimize premature or avoidable dependence on long-term care in institutional settings. The four principles of the National Service Framework for older people – person-centred care, whole system working, timely access to specialist care, and promoting health and active life – should underpin the development of intermediate care services for patients with a hip fracture.

Practicalities relating to the day-to-day provision of services need to be addressed, and professionals working in both acute and community care sectors must work collaboratively to ensure that there is a clear framework for the delivery of intermediate care. Clearly there must be a robust assessment process to identify eligible service users, but, for example, who will assess the patient in order to ensure that the eligibility criteria is met? Will it be the multidisciplinary team involved in caring for the patient since admission to hospital with a hip fracture, or will it be necessary for a member of the intermediate care team to come and further assess the patient? If it is the latter, will there be sufficient staff to respond to referrals in a timely manner, ensuring that transfer to an intermediate care facility is not delayed? If it is the former, will all members of the team have a comprehensive understanding of the intermediate care model of service delivery? Questions such as these need to be answered before any intermediate care service is developed, or there will be a risk of confusion, duplication and fragmentation in the delivery of the service.

Whatever model of intermediate care is adopted, it is essential that a multidisciplinary assessment is undertaken, with the thoughts and wishes of the patient being central to any decision that is made. For those patients requiring rehabilitation following hip fracture there may be inequity in terms of access to any kind of rehabilitation service and with the provision of social care services on discharge home. An acute hospital may provide hip fracture care for patients from a number of primary care trusts. Some of these trusts will have excellent, wide-ranging and well-developed community rehabilitation services, but this is not always the case and not all older people will have access to services required. This is the 'postcode lottery' that has been noticeable in other areas of health care provision (Department of Health 2000b, BBC News 2003). Provision of social services may also vary from area to area, and this may raise questions with reference to the delivery of person-centred care (Standard Two). Patients may remain in hospital longer than they need while awaiting care packages, and in some cases suitable care packages for their individual needs cannot be provided; for example, because of insufficient staff for the delivery of care at home.

Another key element of the National Service Framework is that 'access to long-term residential care should be through intermediate care, hospital rehabilitation and domiciliary or step-down care units to allow opportunities for prevention, treatment, rehabilitation and domiciliary support to be fully explored (before placement is decided upon) and to support patients in making the transition to long-term care' (National Service Framework Standard Four). Care requiring the skills of a qualified nurse will be free of charge when a person is admitted to a care home. For some patients with a hip fracture the prospect of admission to long-term care is a very real one, and both patients and their carers need support and advice in order to assist them through this transitional process.

The National Service Framework for Older People provides a series of specific implementation milestones to help measure the progress made towards the transformation of standards of care and services for older people. The Healthcare Commission, Audit Commission and Commission for Social Care and Inspection are currently undertaking 15 reviews of local communities, and a national report will be published at the end of 2005. Progress will be measured against the standards of the National Service Framework for Older People, so that good practice can be shared and immediate action can be taken where necessary to further improve services (Healthcare Commission 2004). In the care and management of patients with a hip fracture it is important that in order to transform standards of care and services their needs and those of all older people are seen as the top priority. The question that we must ask ourselves is whether or not this is the case.

Reimbursement

As described in previous chapters, timely and effective discharge planning is an integral part of the care of older people with a hip fracture. In 2003 the Community Care (delayed discharges, etc.) Act was introduced. As a result of this act the NHS is required to notify local authorities of any patient's likely need for community care services, and of their proposed discharge date. If a patient has to remain in hospital because the local authority has not arranged the necessary services, it will pay the NHS body a charge per day of delay (DH 2003e). The challenge for acute trusts, primary care trusts and social services departments is to organize discharge for patients with complex health and social care needs promptly. In rising to this challenge delayed discharges will be reduced, reimbursement charges will not be incurred and resources will be used to best effect. The various agencies involved in the care of patients will need to work collaboratively to provide person-centred care, with effective communication being central to improving discharge from hospital and preventing reimbursement charges. The evidence suggests that conflicts between health and social services has been a major barrier to effective discharge planning in the past (McWilliams and Wong 1994). The reasons for some of these conflicts probably relate to the social structures of the organizations, rather than being attributable to individual practitioners, and in order to move towards meeting the ideal of multidisciplinary working, and ensure alliances and effective partnerships across professional boundaries, we need to develop a deeper understanding of the complex dynamics of institutional cultures, professional enculturation and territoriality (Payne et al. 2002). If we are to break down the barriers to communication, we need to attempt to develop an understanding of and respect for each other's roles.

Despite the implementation of the Community Care (delayed discharges) Act, there will clearly still be difficulties in discharging patients from acute hospital environments if the infrastructure is not available to support the needs of some individuals. Some patients who sustain a hip fracture will never fully recover from their injury and will require admission to a continuing care facility. As previously suggested, access to long-term care should be through intermediate care, hospital rehabilitation and domiciliary or step-down care units. Because some of these facilities are not available, many patients continue to wait for placement on acute trauma wards. They may wait a long time, because the lack of non-acute care facilities may also be compounded by delays in access to long-term care facilities because of limited availability.

As the population ages, the demands for long-term care placements will increase, with demographic prediction models highlighting the need for more institutional care. It is predicted that residential places (in residential care homes, nursing homes and hospitals) would need to expand from approximately 450 000 in 2000 to 1 130 000 in 2051, to keep pace with demographic pressures (Wittenberg et al. 2001). It has also been suggested that the number of people with cognitive impairment in institutional care will rise by 63%, from 224 000 in 1998 to 365 000 in 2031 (PSSRU 2003). Although demographic models predict increased demands for long-term beds, concerns have been raised about the fall in the availability of these beds (Bunce 2001,Wanless 2002). The results of a national survey indicated that with the nursing places in nursing and dual registered homes having dropped by 4.9% in a year (31 March 2000–31 March 2001) there is a possibility of an overall reduction in places of 20% within 5 years if this rate of reduction continues (Netten et al. 2003). There is also considerable regional variation in the closure of nursing and dual registered homes, with 7% of nursing homes closing in the south of the country, compared with 3% in the West Midlands and Eastern regions (see Fig. 10.1).

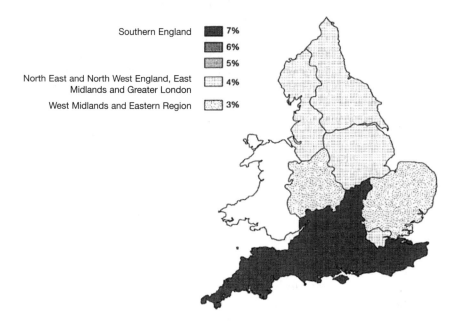

Figure 10.1 Rates of closure of care homes by region, 2000–2001. Source Netten et al (2003) Nursing home closures effects on capacity and reason for closure. Age and Ageing 32: 332–7. Reprinted with kind permission of Oxford University Press.

Reasons for closures and loss of available beds are complex and are often attributable to a range of factors that act in combination, such as:

- Fee levels set by local authorities that are considered to be too low, and low expectations about future fee levels.
- Rising property prices – particularly significant for smaller homes where, because of a combination of low fees and high property prices the care provider may find it more lucrative to sell the property and leave the care home market.
- Problems recruiting managers, qualified nursing staff and basic care staff. In the case of care staff, nursing and care homes are now competing for a pool of people, who with the introduction of the national minimum wage, can work in less demanding jobs than care work for the same wage. With these difficulties in recruitment there is also an underlying concern about the ability of care home providers to deliver a level of care that meets the needs of increasingly dependent clients.

Even with an amendment to the minimum care standards for care homes for older people (DH 2002e), some providers have been unwilling or unable to meet the new standards.

How we address this problem as it continues to escalate is one of the biggest issues facing health and social care providers and policy makers as we evaluate the implementation and impact of key policies and their relation to improving the care of older people. Initiatives that are aimed at preventing dependency and providing greater opportunities for care at home must be applauded, but it cannot be denied that there will be groups of older people who reach a stage where the level of care they require cannot be provided for them at home. It is imperative that their needs are not overlooked, and we must invest in long-term care if we are to prevent a 'complete gridlock of the British hospital service through the overwhelming demand from elderly community refugees seeking asylum in hospitals' (Bowman 2002).

As this chapter has progressed it has become apparent that many policies and reports have an impact on the care that is delivered to the patient with a hip fracture. It could be argued that the implementation of these policies, guidelines and recommendations should considerably improve the care of the patient with a hip fracture, and that care could be standardized and streamlined throughout the NHS. However, we are aware that there are gaps in service delivery and barriers to implementation of policy in clinical practice. It is important to consider reasons for this, because in our failure to implement these guidelines and policies we fall short in the delivery of the service that older people with a hip fracture deserve.

In order to drive up standards and meet policy recommendations, it is essential that we have a workforce adequately trained to meet the needs of older people who are admitted to acute trauma wards. Meeting the educational needs of staff working in daily clinical practice must not be under-estimated. The implementation of policies such as reimbursement requires considerable educational input, in order to ensure that nursing staff have ade-quate knowledge of the philosophy underpinning new policy initiatives, and the practical skills to complete new documentation. Without adequate education of the workforce these policy initiatives are at risk of failure.

In meeting the challenges of improving the care of older people in acute trauma wards, the training of unqualified staff is crucial as they are often providing most of the hands-on care on a day-to-day basis. The Age Concern report *Dignity on the Ward – Promoting Excellence in Care* (HA/RCN 2000) advocated the role of nurse specialists in improving and promoting better care for older people in acute hospital areas. Through role modelling, education, practice development and direct patient care the nurse specialist can work with unqualified as well as trained team mem-bers using influencing skills to assist in the shaping and delivery of care that will improve the patient experience. When working with these staff members, an opportunity can be provided to enable them to reflect on their own attitudes, values and beliefs about older people. Assisting staff to develop self-awareness can facilitate change in their beliefs and attitudes, and this will lead to improvements in the delivery of the fundamental and essential aspects of care.

Not all ward areas will have access to the skills of an older person's spe-cialist nurse, and the role of the ward manager is clearly pivotal in influencing clinical practice, raising standards and ensuring effective care delivery. It is also the responsibility and role of the ward manager to ensure that all staff have appropriate training to undertake their job. Training and knowledge will empower staff with the knowledge and skills required to meet the needs of older patients for whom they care.

In pre-registration education there is now more emphasis on gerontolog-ical education, but it is still not sufficiently addressed (DH 2001h). The result is that newly qualified nurses do not have all the necessary skills and know-ledge to care for older people. Post-registration courses have been developed in gerontology, promoting this as a specialist field of practice within nursing. A key objective for the future is to ensure that enough nurses demonstrate interest in developing expert gerontological skills, when there are many other competing specialisms that may appear more attractive. Raising aware-ness of issues relating to older people and the educational opportunities that are available for nursing staff to enhance their knowledge and skills is essen-tial if we are to ensure that improving the care of older people remains a key objective of nursing in the twenty-first century.

It is apparent that working towards the milestones of the National Service Framework for Older People and the implementation of other major policy recommendations such as those contained in the Community Care

(Delayed Discharges, etc.) Act 2003 demands an enormous amount of energy and commitment from all stakeholders and practitioners involved in the implementation process, as we strive to improve the experience of older people with a hip fracture. Strong leadership and a shared vision of rooting out age discrimination, providing person-centred care and improving the whole experience of the older person is essential if we are to progress towards transforming policy rhetoric into clinical practice. Although there needs to be a commitment to meeting shared goals at every level within the NHS organization, there are key players who can lead in the transformation of the care that we deliver to older patients with a hip fracture.

In 2001, modern matrons were introduced as part of the NHS Plan (DH 2001g, 2002d, 2003f). The Health Service circular described the matron as 'a strong clinical leader with clear authority at ward level who is highly visible, accessible and easily identifiable by patients and has real authority to ensure the basics of care are met'. The 10 things that modern matrons do have been identified as:

- Lead by example – by demonstrating to other nurses the high standards of care NHS patients can expect.
- Make sure patients get quality care – by taking responsibility for driving up standards of care and leading work to improve professional practice and patient services.
- Make sure wards are clean – by setting and monitoring standards and taking action to ensure specifications are met.
- Ensure patients' nutritional needs are met – by ensuring that patients get the right meals, at the right time, and that they are able to eat them.
- Prevent hospital-acquired infection – by ensuring that infection control measures are properly applied by all staff
- Improve the ward for patients – by overseeing spending of ward environment budgets by ward sisters and charge nurses.
- Empower nurses – by enabling more nurses to undertake a wider range of clinical responsibilities to speed up patient care, such as admitting and discharging patients, ordering tests and prescribing medicines.
- Make sure patients are treated with respect – by ensuring their privacy and dignity are protected and making sure they are addressed in the way they choose.
- Resolve problems for patients and their relatives – by acting quickly to deal with problems when and where they occur and working closely with the patient advice and liaison service.
- Ensuring staffing is appropriate to patient need – by working with ward sisters and charge nurses to assess patient dependency and adjust duty rosters, and to develop proposals for changes to skill mix and staff establishments.

Looking at this list, it is noticeable that these responsibilities are clearly linked to the Essence of Care. It can be argued that in their pivotal role matrons help to inject a renewed interest in the fundamental and essential aspects of care, using the benchmarking tool as an aid to encourage professional staff to question their practice, and drive up standards towards improving the quality of the patient experience. Matrons are at the forefront of the modernization of the NHS, and are key players in improving the patient experience.

The first milestones in the National Service Framework for Older People included the appointment of champions for older people, who would be key players in local programmes to modernize health and social services (DH 2001a, p. 18). For each local health and social care system there should be:

- an elected member or an NHS non-executive director who will lead for older people across each organization
- a clinical or practice champion within each organization to lead professional development
- in NHS trusts, an older people's patient champion through the patient's forum to look after patient interests.

The role of champions for older people is crucial in maintaining the momentum for implementing the National Service Framework for Older People and supporting the involvement of older people at a local level. In recognizing the pivotal role of these champions for older people, Age Concern developed a champion's pledge with older people, which was launched in June 2001. It focused on three key principles where champions can support the successful implementation of the National Service Framework. These are:

- to challenge ageist attitudes and promote respect for older people
- to engage and involve older people, listen and learn from their experiences
- to respect the diversity of older people and encourage cultural sensitivity (Age Concern 2002).

Clearly the challenges for older people's champions are great, and anyone who undertakes this as just one part of their job may at times find it almost impossible to give sufficient time to the role and meet the expectations of the National Service Framework. Findings from a survey of 209 older people's champions (BGOP 2003) highlighted how they are not always clear about what is expected of them, or how to influence or take the lead on change. Most see their role as a way of raising the profile of older people's services and maintaining the momentum of the National

Service Framework for Older People. What patients, carers and health care professionals want to know is if they are making a difference.

Over many years we have witnessed a proliferation of new nursing roles in the NHS, partly influenced in some by health and social care policy reform. One of the most recent role developments has been that of consultant nurse, supporting and recognizing the importance of clinical career pathways for nurses who want to follow a career structure that enables them to contribute to meeting the health needs of the population while promoting health gain (DH 1999). Clear expectations of the role of consultant nurses have been identified and incorporate four key functions:

- expert practice function
- education, training and development function
- practice and service development, research and evaluation function
- professional leadership and consultancy function (NHSE 1999).

These core functions have been defined by the Department of Health, but there has been considerable flexibility for NHS trusts in developing posts to shape and meet the needs of the local population. For the role of a consultant nurse for older people, for example, boundaries would need to be established as otherwise the scope of the role might be too wide, and it is clear that the role could be developed in a number of directions dependent upon local priorities. In encompassing the four elements of their role, consultant nurses are working towards advancing the art and science of practice in their chosen field (Redfern 2003). In the care of older people, they are in particularly strong positions to challenge practice at every level. Such roles can be considered as key drivers for the successful implementation of policy initiatives that affect the care that we deliver to older people.

A common link running through all of the above-mentioned roles is the need for strong leadership skills. Strong leadership and change management skills are essential if we are to assist health care professionals at every level to engage in positive actions which will ensure that policies, guidelines and recommendations are put into operation. Having raised the profile of older people and their experiences of acute health care delivery, we must ensure that improving the quality of care that they receive, in whatever health or social care setting, remains at the very top of our agenda.

CHAPTER ELEVEN

Future developments

In our quest to gain a better understanding of the epidemiology, prevention and management of hip fractures many challenges have become apparent – challenges that need our urgent attention as we face the predicted rise in hip fractures worldwide (Ahranonoff et al. 1997). In rising to these challenges it must be acknowledged that we simply cannot do more of the same but must rethink the way that we provide hip fracture care, ensuring that we have the right people at all levels in the organization who are adequately equipped to meet the demands facing us. These challenges include:

- reduction of high mortality rates that are associated with hip fracture
- development of multidisciplinary falls services that incorporate the diagnosis and management of osteoporosis
- development and recommendation of evidence-based hip fracture care programmes that encompass all aspects of care
- provision of responsive rehabilitation programmes
- provision of long-term care beds in response to predicted future demands
- production and evaluation of new surgical approaches to hip fracture care.

In considering these challenges it could be argued that the best way to prevent mortality rates associated with hip fracture is early identification of fracture risk and implementation of preventive measures. Evidence suggests that a previous low-energy fracture is among the strongest risk factors for new fractures (Nevitt et al. 1999, Cummings and Melton 2002): individuals with a prior vertebral fracture have an up to sixfold increased risk of hip and other non-vertebral fractures compared to individuals with no history of fracture (Gunnes et al. 1998, van Staa et al. 2002b). Clinical trials have demonstrated that treatment of fragility fractures can reduce the risk of future fractures by up to 50% (Hochberg 2000, Delmas 2002). These findings support the imperative of optimizing the care of patients with fragility fractures.

185

How, then, do we optimize the care of people with fragility fractures, and in so doing reduce the risk of hip fracture? As previously suggested, osteoporosis is generally a silent disease until a person presents with a fracture, and general population screening is not currently recommended. When reviewing patients in fracture clinics, orthopaedic surgeons are in a unique position to consider osteoporosis as a possible antecedent to the presenting fracture, educate the fracture patient about the need to decrease the risk for future fractures, initiate investigations and make appropriate referrals for further follow-up as required. It can be argued that orthopaedic surgeons are now more aware of the role of osteoporosis in the genesis of hip fracture and are therefore better equipped in terms of knowledge to take an active role in managing or referring patients with fragility fractures. However, poor referral rates for DXA scans from orthopaedic outpatient clinics have been identified (Eastell et al. 2001) and most orthopaedic surgeons do not see the need to investigate or treat osteoporosis in patients presenting with hip fracture (Sheehan et al. 2000).

Bearing this in mind, along with the difficult problem of time management in busy fracture clinics, it seems that the establishment of a fracture liaison service could offer the best solution in terms of the management of fragility fracture patients who attend fracture clinics. Specialist nurses could take the lead in the initiation of such a service with support and access to physicians specializing in the management of metabolic bone disease as required according to locally developed protocols. On trauma wards the older person's specialist nurse could also take a lead role in the care, education and management of patients with fragility fractures. In the development of such services all members of the multidisciplinary team need to have the motivation, drive and desire to effectively implement change in order to successfully provide services and improve the care delivered to patients with fragility fractures. Protocols and guidelines will also need to be developed to include:

* identification of those patients at risk
* rationale and consideration of patients appropriate for bone densitometry.
* bone health promotion
* interpretation of DXA scan results
* treatment guidelines
* referral guidelines for specialist follow-up.

As with any service development, a cost–benefit analysis needs to be undertaken and once developed the service needs to be analysed in terms of:

* patients' level of satisfaction with the service
* patients' understanding of osteoporosis and its management

- referral rates for investigations
- costs of investigations and prescribing costs
- referring clinicians' level of satisfaction with the service.

As identified in Chapter 2, there are still many areas within the epidemiology, investigation and treatment of osteoporosis that provide conflicting evidence, making it more challenging to advocate the development of such services, particularly as the results of their implementation may not be apparent for several years. However, taking into account the high personal costs to individuals who sustain a hip fracture and the financial burden in terms of health and social care costs associated with fragility fractures (Torgerson et al. 2001), it is essential that health professionals take an active role in managing patients with fragility fractures in order to 'substantially improve the long-term outcome of these patients, reduce the risk of subsequent fracture, and thereby help mitigate the downward spiral in health and quality of life that often follows fractures' (AAOS 2004). Although healthcare professionals take a key role in the development and management of services, improved fracture care within our communities needs to be supported by local acute and primary care trusts and national government if we are going to make any progress in reducing the predicted increase in numbers of people sustaining a hip fracture.

In the prevention and management of fragility fracture we also have an increasing body of evidence that points to falls prevention strategies that can be utilized in our attempts to reduce the incidence of hip fracture. The development of an integrated falls service in all primary care trusts is a key milestone of Standard Six of the National Services Framework for older people (DH 2001a). Several key factors are necessary for the successful implementation of a falls prevention programme. These have been discussed in Chapter 3, but it is now worth recapping the salient points that emerged from that discussion.

Assessment

Assessment of older people at risk of falling is an integral part of any falls prevention strategy, with the intensity of that assessment being tailored to the target population. In the community, all older people should be asked at least once a year about falls. Those in high risk groups such as those who are unsteady when they stand, those who have experienced more than two falls in a year and those in institutional care settings require a detailed and comprehensive assessment. Any older patient admitted to a trauma ward with a fragility fracture should also have a comprehensive assessment. The use of a valid and reliable assessment tool, which is easy to use and applicable to the particular setting in which it is being used, can assist in making an objective and systematic assessment easier.

Investigation of the principal cause of the fall

In assessing the person who has fallen it is important to obtain a thorough history of the fall taking into account a description of activities being undertaken at the time of the fall, symptoms such as dizziness or legs giving way that were experienced prior to or at the time of the fall, and any previous history of falls. Some individuals may experience difficulty in recalling the events leading up to, and the circumstances of the fall. In these situations, reports from witnesses should be obtained whenever possible.

Assessment and investigation of the principal cause of the fall using a risk factor-based approach can prevent more than 50% of falls (Close 2001). In order to undertake a comprehensive assessment, it is essential that professionals have an underpinning knowledge of at-risk patients and possible environmental, intrinsic and extrinsic risk factors that can contribute to a fall. It has been suggested that the skill of the professional undertaking the risk assessment is more important than the effectiveness of the risk assessment tool in the efficacy of falls risk assessment (Willis 1998) and the development of a care plan that is used with an assessment tool is an example of best practice (Kelly and Dowling 2004).

Implementation of falls prevention strategies

Assessment and investigation of the principal cause of the fall can assist us in identifying those patients who would benefit from a falls prevention programme. Many strategies have been identified for use with community-dwelling older people, those living in institutional care and patients in acute care environments. Many factors contribute to the risk of falling and cause falls, so it is perhaps therefore not surprising that evidence supports targeted multifactorial interventions as likely to be the most successful in any falls prevention programme (Shaw and Kenny 1998, Sullivan and Badros 1999). A multifactorial approach is important because it is not possible to tell which of the multifactorial interventions are the most effective (Chang et al. 2004).

Properly targeted falls prevention strategies can help in reducing falls and subsequent hip fracture. However, despite the association between risk of falling and dementia there is little evidence to demonstrate the effectiveness of prevention strategies in reducing the number of falls in this group. Given the number of patients who present with a hip fracture and have cognitive impairment, it is necessary to consider other strategies that can be utilized in reducing the risk to this particularly vulnerable group. In recent years attention has been drawn to the use of hip protectors as a means of reducing the number of hip fractures, and results from various studies have been promising (Chan et al. 2000, Harada et al. 2001, Parker et al. 2005).

It could be argued that in an attempt to reduce the incidence of hip fracture, hip protector pants should be provided to all nursing home residents. However, before implementing such a strategy we must take into account other factors, unrelated to the efficacy of the appliance, that have an impact upon the effectiveness of hip protectors. Dementia has been the most significant factor identified in low patient acceptability and adherence with the wearing of hip protector pants (Chan et al. 2000). This is significant, when we consider that other falls prevention strategies do not appear to reduce the risk of falls in this particular group. Adherence and low patient acceptability may be related to the fact that hip protectors need to be worn 24 hours a day, are made of polypropylene and are uncomfortable because of their weight. Improvements have been made in the design of hip protectors, but adherence will remain the single most important barrier to achieving maximal benefit (O'Toole 2002). Evidence also suggests that wearing hip protectors does not always prevent hip fracture in the event of a fall (Meyer et al. 2003, O'Halloran et al. 2004). They should only be used in combination with an education programme for nursing staff, other caregivers and if possible, the people who will be wearing them (Meyer et al. 2003). It has been argued that until 'more efficacious hip protectors are available, and until more is known about how adherence to their use can be improved, health care commissioners should not provide hip protectors free of charge to all nursing home residents' (O'Halloran et al. 2004).

The evidence that supports falls and fracture prevention is growing, and although some areas will benefit from further research and development there is no doubt that a comprehensive falls prevention strategy, which includes the prevention and management of osteoporosis, will have a considerable impact on future hip fracture incidence. However, even when such strategies are implemented there will still be significant numbers of older people who present with hip fracture, and in these situations our primary aim should be to enhance the care they receive.

Hip fractures in the older population have serious implications for both mortality and morbidity, as well as significant impacts on health and social services utilization. When we consider the care of the patient with a hip fracture there is a growing body of evidence that should enable us to practice evidence-based care; however, barriers, including gaps in current knowledge, do exist and these can prevent the delivery of best practice. In

Scotland the surgical element of hip fracture is already well audited (Scottish National Hip Fracture Audit) and there are various regional UK audits. Currently, the British Orthopaedic Association, the British Geriatric Society and the Royal College of Physicians (London) have taken the first steps towards the development of an audit tool for hip fracture that also incorporates standards for falls risk and bone health. Orthogeriatric input and care will also be evaluated.

Hip fracture is well recognized as a sentinel event, it is easily defined and primarily affects a population that can also be readily identified. These factors should facilitate reliable and valid audit. In undertaking such a large-scale audit, it is important to recognize that audit by itself will not lead to improved patient care. However, in the case of stroke – which offers a similar model in the care of older people – the National Sentinel audit, based on well-established evidence-based guidelines relating to the organization of services, appropriate clinical management of stroke patients, including the need for secondary prevention and outcomes of care, has been successful in highlighting the variation and limitations in stroke care around the country (RCP 2004). Similar deficits have been highlighted in the audit on myocardial infarction (RCP 2003) and these audits have been instrumental in service developments in many trusts.

It has been argued that hip fracture, orthogeriatric rehabilitation and associated secondary prevention in terms of falls and bone health are analogous to stroke services (BGS 2004) with a substantial evidence base to guide best practice. In developing a hip fracture audit there will be a more comprehensive evaluation of service provision to older people who fall, with deficits in care being highlighted. These factors will act as a driving force in raising standards of care and shaping future services in the care for older people who fall and sustain a hip fracture. Furthermore, hip fracture audit will enable us to meet the requirements of the National Service Framework to develop indicators for falls services.

In sharing a commitment to working together, the British Geriatric Society (BGS) and British Orthopaedic Association (BOA) can use a combined approach to improve the care of patients with fragility fractures. In working collaboratively new opportunities will arise with areas for future developments including a joint research agenda, health service evaluation/implementation and a combined approach to the training of future consultants in orthopaedic surgery and geriatric medicine (BOA/BGS 2004). Clearly, it is also important to ensure that nurses and other allied health care professionals are included in the development of services and practice innovations in our quest to improve the care of older people with fragility fractures. With a combined approach and a shared vision of raising standards of care for this patient population change can be facilitated nationally in the political, clinical, educational and academic arenas.

The development of a national hip fracture audit in England is to be applauded, but as previously suggested it will not in itself lead to improved care but will act as a powerful driver for change and assist in ensuring the effective and efficient targeting of resources.

For those older people who sustain a hip fracture, time to surgery is a key indicator in terms of morbidity and mortality. Many surgical delays can be fundamentally linked to a lack of resources in terms of personnel or infrastructure, and an urgent reallocation of resources is needed to address this issue. Health care practitioners caring for this group of patients must be prepared to lobby and challenge current resource allocation as investment in terms of reducing delays to surgery could be recouped by reducing the number of bed days and the use of other resources that often occur as a result of delays in surgery. Achievable benchmarks in terms of time to surgery need to be established (e.g. 90% of patients operated on within 24 hours) as a quality indicator at local level to ensure that timely surgical intervention occurs and to measure the end result of any resource re-allocation.

The surgical management of hip fractures offers many challenges to the orthopaedic surgeon, with the long-term functional consequences of fracture being dependent on surgical success, as much in the care of hip fracture patients as in any other group (BOA 2003). Current surgical techniques for the fixation of hip fracture, while successful in repairing the fracture itself, often damage surrounding muscles and tissues. Because the initial surgical incision involves cutting through muscle and soft tissue, the leg is substantially weakened, causing instability that can often result in lengthy rehabilitation times with four out of five patients having a decline in ambulatory status (Audit Commission 1995, 2000, SIGN 2002). Other serious complications from surgery can also arise, largely due to the patients' decreased level of activity.

An innovative new approach to hip fracture treatment aims to provide fixation and controlled reduction of all types of hip fracture through a minimally invasive technique. Minimally invasive surgery with an incision of only 2.5–5 cm, avoids the need to cut through the muscle nerves and blood vessels. If this is used in conjunction with new implant devices, the need for dissection of much of the area around the ball and socket joint is avoided. This innovative surgical technique should ensure that the stability and strength of the leg is maintained, significantly reduce surgical recovery time, increase mobility immediately after the surgery, decrease rehabilitation time and offer a greater chance of resuming a normal level of activity after surgery, which, in turn, will decrease the risk of pulmonary and other complications (Notre Dame 2002).

Minimally invasive techniques should contribute significantly to the improved management of the patient with a hip fracture, particularly in relation to early rehabilitation and the achievement of maximal functional outcome in a shorter period of time. On a more cautionary note, it is important to recognize that the impact of minimally invasive surgery on infection and venous thromboembolism rates is not clearly established (Kwong 2003) and it is therefore necessary to ensure that established protocols in relation to antibiotic and thromboembolic prophylaxis are merged with developing technology.

It has also been suggested that technical aspects of hip fracture fixation could be improved. One method of enhancing stability involves the injection of polymethyl-methacrylate (to solidify fixation) into or around a fracture site, and then putting a screw or other form of fixation into the bone resulting in a more stable fixation, reduction in pain and restoration of function (Kramer et al. 2000, Larsson and Bauer 2002). Current research is focusing on a procedure known as femoroplasty-augmentation, with the suggestion that prophylactic reinforcement of the femur could become a treatment option to solve the problems associated with osteoporotic hip fracture in patients at risk (Heini et al. 2004).

Areas for further research in the surgical management of the patient with a hip fracture include new surgical methods such as implants designed specifically for osteoporotic bone and implants modified to produce biological stimuli at the site of the repair (BOA 2003).

Innovative surgical techniques will contribute positively to improvements in hip fracture care. As well as these new surgical approaches, evidence-based recommendations encompassing all aspects of care should form the basis of hip fracture care programmes. We already have a considerable body of evidence supporting current guidelines in the care of hip fracture patients (Audit Commission 1995, 2000, SIGN 2002). The challenge now is to ensure that these guidelines are fully integrated into clinical practice and that research is undertaken in those areas where gaps in knowledge exist.

As we move forward in the development of hip fracture care, it is important to recognize the fundamental importance of cooperation between orthopaedic surgeons and geriatricians in the management of patients with fragility fractures. This cooperation should move beyond rehabilitation and must also encompass multidisciplinary perioperative care (NCEPOD 1999, Sharrock 2000, Marsh 2003). As mentioned earlier, there are four models of orthogeriatric care currently in use in England and the model which is adopted depends on local resources. The model supported by the BOA is that of combined orthogeriatric care with a medical consultant or staff-grade physician working full time on the fracture ward. In 2003 a study of orthogeriatric liaison services in England demonstrated that only four departments had the model of care highlighted above (Wakeman et al. 2004). These findings highlighted the difficulty of ensuring the presence of a daytime physician, with insufficient clinicians with appropriate training being available to fill potential vacancies. However, hospital trusts can be creative with the resources that they have at their disposal and models of orthogeriatric liaison can be adapted to meet local needs, as for example, in the model described in Chapter 8. Whatever model of orthogeriatric liaison is utilized, the overarching aim is to improve the standard of care for older people with hip fractures. An orthogeriatric liaison service allows for:

- early identification and treatment of complications with a reduction in adverse events
- optimal scheduling of operations on the fractures
- better communication with patient, relatives and the multidisciplinary team
- facilitation of research, education and audit
- earlier initiation of rehabilitation
- more effective use of resources for discharge.

Effective rehabilitation is essential if we are to improve morbidity and mortality rates associated with hip fracture. It has been suggested that the primary goal of geriatric rehabilitation is to improve abilities in all activities of daily living, ranging from eating to managing finances (Röder et al. 2003). In achieving these goals it is important not only to focus on functional and physical mobility but to use a more holistic approach that includes the social, psychological and emotional health of individual patients. In the case of patients with a hip fracture, different approaches for inpatient rehabilitation have been recommended but clinical outcomes are heterogeneous (Johnson et al. 2000, Cree et al. 2001). Some authors have argued that patients who are transferred to rehabilitation units will gain higher functional scores. However, a recent study found no data to support the expectation that rehabilitation in orthopaedic or geriatric hospitals had a major impact on the clinical outcome in the population tested (Röder et al. 2003), and in a Cochrane review no statistically significant better outcome for patients with proximal femoral fractures receiving coordinated inpatient rehabilitation was found in the literature (Cameron et al. 2000). Such findings obviously have implications for the rehabilitation of patients with hip fracture, and patients clearly need to be stratified into those who can be discharged directly home and those who need and would benefit from inpatient rehabilitation. In order to make the appropriate decisions for an individual patient prognostic characteristics such as dementia, prefracture fitness and health, postoperative complications and undernutrition, which have all been identified as factors associated with poor functional outcome, need to be taken into consideration. Again, the role of the experts in the care of older people is significant in assisting orthopaedic surgeons in making decisions about patients who would most benefit from rehabilitation. More research also needs to be undertaken into the role of rehabilitation and its impact on clinical outcomes in the care of older patients with a hip fracture.

In the care of a patient with a hip fracture who also has cognitive impairment there are many areas of concern. As previously highlighted, falls prevention strategies that have proved successful with other older people do not appear to have the same effect when used in people with cognitive impairment. Problems with concordance in the use of hip protector pants have also been highlighted as being particularly prevalent in people with cognitive impairment. Given these factors it appears that individuals with cognitive impairment will continue to present with hip fracture and as the population ages it is clear that significant costs will be incurred in relation to health and social care for this group of patients.

In considering rehabilitation strategies it is important that we do not deny rehabilitation for this group of patients, and the avoidance of disability through appropriate rehabilitation should remain a priority. However, despite these strategies it is also apparent that many of these patients are less likely to return to independent living. Reasons for this are multifactorial, and even with intensive rehabilitation the person may remain too disabled to live at home independently. Resources may not be available to cope with managing a dependent person with dementia at home. It could be argued that this is unacceptable in this age of patient choice and increased respect for autonomy, but the reality is that support at home requiring more than 4 hours of care a day is more expensive than care home placement, and support at night is very hard to come by. Thus, intensive home care for this group of patients is extremely difficult to provide. Consideration also has to be given to informal 'caregivers', who may find the strain of caring for a person with progressive dementia and its attendant symptoms such as poor safety awareness, fluctuating need for assistance and 24 hour need for supervision burdensome in terms of their own health and well-being. While recognizing the need to increase the number of choices available to patients and their families, it must be recognized that not all placements will be avoidable.

In a recent national census of care home residents it was clearly demonstrated that dementia, stroke and other neurodegenerative diseases with mental impairment were the major determining factors leading to admission to long-term care, with the suggestion that it is unlikely that the needs of the people with these levels of dependency could in practice be met in the community (Bowman et al. 2004).

In future care commissioning, urgent attention must be given to the loss of 60 000 care home beds in the UK over the past 5 years (Ellerby 2003) and the possible consequences in terms of care of older people and the impact on acute hospital services (Bowman 2002). A further challenge for commissioners and providers is the development of a new long-term care strategy that encapsulates the provision of care to a subset of older people who have complex needs that cannot be met through preventative strategies and various forms of community care. Care home commissioning currently reflects a social model of care. Given the reasons identified for admission to institutional care, it is apparent that a different model needs to be adopted in order to address the health and social care needs of older people requiring admission to institutional care. The distinction between nursing and residential categories has been questioned, and needs further exploration (Rothera et al. 2003, Bowman et al. 2004). Person-centred care can only be adequately provided to care home residents if there is better management of the health/social interface with particular attention being paid to balancing the need for provision of medical care, rehabilitation, occupation, personal and nursing care.

Person-centred care for older people should be at the core of the service that we deliver in the care of the patient with a hip fracture. In demonstrating respect for, value of and promotion of personhood, therapeutic relationships can be developed between professionals and the patients that they care for, ensuring that the focus is on individuals and their perception of the situation they are in. In utilizing this approach in clinical practice we can move towards improving the experience of patients and their care. Audit of hip fracture care is important not only in terms of length of stay in the Accident and Emergency department, time to surgery, and length of stay but also in terms of the level of care that patients experience on a daily basis. The 'Essence of Care' can assist us in measuring the quality of care that we deliver, highlighting gaps in care delivery and enabling us to share in our successes and drive up standards throughout an organization. As previously suggested, patient narratives and observations of care are also powerful tools at our disposal that can be used to inform and improve our practice. They enable us to analyse our practice, contribute to quality assurance, clinical effectiveness and clinical audit, and can therefore contribute significantly to the clinical governance agenda and help us to 'create an environment in which clinical excellence will flourish' (DH 1998a).

As discussed in the previous chapter, in order to ensure that progress is made in the prevention and management of fragility fractures, the need for strong leadership at every level of the NHS organization cannot be underestimated. It is through strong leadership that challenges to the process can be made and a shared vision can be inspired. Government commitment through investment in and education of future leaders needs to be continued. Joint initiatives between professional organizations such as those between the BOA and BGS will do much to help progress future developments in the care of patients with fragility fractures.

In responding to service demands and the need for effective service delivery there is an urgent need to review current models of service delivery. This should include a review of traditional roles within the multidisciplinary team and an exploration of how current roles can be enhanced and developed to ensure that innovative and responsive practice is developed to meet the needs of the older patient with a hip fracture. For example, consideration might be given to the development of a consultant practitioner role within the field of orthogeriatrics. The consultant practitioner could act as a driver for the development and delivery of responsive services that include the prevention as well as the management of hip fractures. As previously suggested, the model of service delivery will be dependent upon local needs, but with the growing body of evidence available in relation to hip fracture prevention and management, it is essential that the key elements as identified in the introduction to this chapter are incorporated into future service delivery plans.

In improving our approaches to the prevention of hip fractures and ensuring that evidence-based care is delivered to patients admitted with this injury, my hope is that in the future fewer of them will 'come into the world through the brim of the pelvis and go out through the neck of the femur'.

Useful websites

Alzheimer's Society *www.alzheimers.org.uk*
British Geriatric Society *www.bgs.org.uk*
British Orthopaedic Association *www.boa.ac.uk*
Help the Aged *www.helptheaged.org.uk*
National Osteoporosis Society *www.nos.org.uk*
National Service Framework *www.dh.gov.uk/PolicyAndGuidance/HealthAndSocialCare
    Topics/OlderPeoplesServices/fs/en*
Nice Guidelines *www.nice.org.uk*
Scottish Intercollegiate Guidelines Network *www.sign.ac.uk/guidelines/fulltext/56*

References

AAOS (2004) Position Statement. Recommendations for enhancing the care of patients with fragility fractures. www.aaos.org/wordhtml/papers/position/1159.htm.

Abdelhafiz AH, Austin CA (2003) Visual factors should be assessed in older people presenting with falls or hip fracture. Age and Ageing 32: 26–30.

ACS (1997) Advanced Trauma Life Support Manual. American College of Surgeons, Chicago, IL.

Age Concern (2002) Champions for Older People: a Briefing from Age Concern. Policy Unit, Age Concern, London.

AGS (2002) American Geriatric Society Panel on persistent pain in older persons. The management of persistent pain in older persons. Journal of the American Geriatric Society 50(6): S205–S224.

AGS/BGS/AAOP (2001) American Geriatric Society, British Geriatric Society and American Academy of Orthopaedic Surgeons Panel on Falls Prevention. Guidelines for the prevention of falls in older people. Journal of the American Geriatric Society 49: 664–72.

Aguero-Torres H, Fratiglioni L, Guo Z, Viitanen M (1998) Dementia is a major cause of dependence in the elderly. 3-year follow-up data from a population-based study. American Journal of Public Health 88(10): 1452–56.

Aharonoff GB, Koval KJ, Skovron ML, Zuckermam JD (1997) Hip fractures in the elderly: predictors of one year mortality. Journal of Orthopaedic Trauma 11: 162–5.

Ahern J, Philpot P (2002) Assessing acutely ill patients on general wards. Nursing Standard 16: 47–54.

All Party Parliamentary Osteoporosis Group (2004) Falling Short: Delivering Integrated Falls and Osteoporosis Services in England. A report on the implementation of Standard Six of the National Service Framework for Older People. All Party Parliamentary Osteoporosis Group, London.

Allen D (2000) The NHS is in need of strong leadership. Nursing Standard 14: 25.

Alonso CG, Curiel MD, Carranza FH, Cano RP, Perez AD (2000) Femoral bone mineral density, neck-shaft angle and mean femoral neck width as predictors of hip fracture in men and women. Multicenter Project for Research in Osteoporosis. Osteoporosis International 11: 714–20.

AMA (2001) Osteoporosis prevention, diagnosis and therapy. JAMA 285(6): 785–995.

Anwar MM (1999) The fracture of the neck of the femur. A review of the relevant aspects as a guide in clinical practice. www.orion-group.net/orion20medical/journal/vo2.Jan.1999.htm.APA (1994) Diagnostic and Statistical Manual of Mental Disorders, 4th edn. American Psychiatric Association, Washington, D.C.

Arnadottir SA, Mercer VS (2000) Effects of footwear on measurements of balance and gait in women between the ages of 65 and 93 years. Physical Therapy 80: 17–27.

Audit Commission (1995) United They Stand: Coordinating Care for Elderly Patients with Hip Fracture. HMSO, London.

Audit Commission (2000) The Way to Go Home. Rehabilitation and Remedial Services for Older People. Audit Commission, London.

Audit Commission (2001) Acute Hospital Portfolio: Review of National Findings – Catering. Audit Commission, London.

Avenell A, Handoll HHG (2004) Nutritional supplementation for hip fracture aftercare in the elderly. (Cochrane review). In The Cochrane Library Issue 2.

Balasegaram S, Majeed A, Fitz-Clarence H (2001) Trends in hospital admissions for fractures of the hip and femur in England, 1989–1990 to 1997–1998. Journal of Public Health Medicine 23: 11–17.

Bandolier (1999) Risk factors for hip fracture in women. www.jr2.ox.ac.uk/bandolier/band66/b66-4.html. August 1999: 66–9.

Barnett JA, Baron J, Karagas MR, Beach ML (1999) Fracture risk in the US Medicare population. Journal of Clinical Epidemiology 52: 243–9.

Baron JA, Farahmand BY, Weierpass E et al. (2001) Cigarette smoking, alcohol consumption and risk of hip fracture in women. Archives of Internal Medicine 161(7): 983–8.

Barr H (2000) New NHS, New collaborative, New agenda for education. Journal of Interprofessional Care 14(1): 81–6.

Baudoin C, Fardelloni P, Potard V, Sekert JL (1993) Fractures of the proximal femur in Picardy, France in 1987. Osteoporosis International 3(1): 43–9.

BBC News (2003) Cancer drug lottery to be tackled. 28 October 2003.

Beaver K, Luker K (1997) Readability of patient information booklets for women with breast cancer. Patient Education and Counselling 31(2): 95–102.

Belbin RMC (1998) Team Roles at Work. Butterworth-Heinemann, Oxford.

Bender M (2003) Explorations in Dementia: Theoretical and Research Studies into the Experience of Remediable and Enduring Cognitive Losses. Jessica Kingsley Publishers, London.

Benesh L, Szigeti E, Ferraro R, Gullicks JN (1997) Tools for assessing chronic pain in rural elderly women. Home Healthcare Nurse 15(3): 207–11.

Benner P (1984) From Novice to Expert: Excellence and Power in Clinical Nursing Practice. Addison-Wesley, Menlo Park, CA.

Benner P, Tanner C, Chelsea C (1996) Expertise in nursing Practice: Caring, Clinical Judgement and Ethics. Springer, New York.

Berge SJ, Morrow-Howell N, Proctor EK (1994) Hip fracture. Clinical Geriatric Medicine 10: 589–609.

BGOP (2003) Better Government for Older People Research Series: No.1. King's College, London.

BGS (2003) Advice on nutrition in common clinical situations. Compendium document G.1. British Geriatric Society, London.

BGS (2004) The discharge of elderly persons from hospital to community care. A joint statement issued by the British Geriatric Society, Association of Directors of Social Services and the Royal College of Nursing. www.bgs.bgs.org.uk.

BGS/RCN (2001) Older person's specialist nurse – a joint statement. British Geriatric Society and the Royal College of Nursing, London.

Biley A (2002) National Service Framework for Older People: promoting health. British Journal of Nursing 11(7): 469–76.

Bird J (2003) Selection of pain measurement tools. Nursing Standard 18(13): 33–9.

Black DM, Steinbuch M, Palermo L, Dargent-Molina P et al. (2001) An assessment tool for predicting fracture risk in postmenopausal women. Osteoporosis International 12: 519–28.

Blake AJ, Morgan K, Bendall MJ, Dollosso H et al. (1998) Falls by elderly people at home: prevalence and associated risk factors. Age and Ageing 17: 365–72.

Blundell CM, Parker MJ, Pryor GA, Hopkinson-Wooley J, Bhousle SS (1998) Assessment of the AO classification of intracapsular fractures of the proximal femur. Journal of Bone and Joint Surgery 80B: 678–83.

BMA (2001) Withholding and Withdrawing Life Prolonging Medical Treatment: Guidance for Decision Making. British Medical Association, London

BNF (2001) Ten Key Facts: Nutrition in Older People. British Nutrition Foundation, London.

BOA (2003) The Care of Fragility Fracture Patients. British Orthopaedic Association, London.

BOA/BGS (2004) A combined approach to fragility fractures. Meeting, British Orthopaedic Association and British Geriatric Society, 12–13 October 2004, London.

Bonjour J-P, Ammann P, Chevalley T, Ferrari C, Rizzoli R (2003) Nutritional aspects of bone growth: an overview. Chapter 3 in New A, Bonjour J-P (eds), Nutritional Aspects of Bone Health. Royal Society of Chemistry, Cambridge.

Bowling A, Grundy E (1997) Activities of daily living: change in functional ability in three samples of elderly and very elderly people. Age and Ageing 26: 107–114.

Bowman C (2003) The new imperative of long-term care. Age and Ageing 32: 246–7.

Bowman C, Whistler J, Ellerby M (2004) A national census of care home residents. Age and Ageing 33: 561–6.

Braden BJ, Bergstron N (1989) Clinical utility of the Braden scale for predicting pressure sore risk. Decubitus 2(3): 44–51.

Bradley L, Rees C (2003) Reducing nutritional risk in hospital: the red tray. Nursing Standard 17(26): 33–7.

Briggs E (2003) The nursing management of pain in older people. Nursing Standard 17(18): 47–53.

Browne GJ, McCaskill ME, Fasher BJ, Lam LT (2001) The benefits of using clinical pathways for managing acute paediatric illness in an emergency department. Journal of Qualitative Clinical Practice 21: 50–5.

Bruce A, Kopp P (2001) Pain experienced by older people. Professional Nurse 16(11): 1481–5.

Buchner DN, Cress ME, Lateur BJ et al. (1997) Strength and endurance training on gait, balance, fall risk and health service use in community living older adults. Journal of Gerontology 52A: M218–M224.

Bunce C (2001) The care home catastrophe. Nursing Times 97: 22–4.

Burns L, Ashwell M, Berry J, Bolton-Smith C et al. (2003) UK Food Standards Agency Optimal Nutrition Status Workshop. Environmental factors that affect bone health throughout life. British Journal of Nutrition 89: 835–40.

Bush T (2003) Communicating with patients who have dementia. Nursing Times 99(48). www.nursingtimes.net/new?page=nt.print&resource=687194.

Butler K, Roche-Tarny D (2002) Succession planning: putting an organisation's knowledge to work. Nature Biotechnology 20(2): 201–2.

Butler M, Norton R, Lieu Joe T, Cheng A, Campbell A (1996) The risk of hip fracture in older people from private homes and institutions. Age and Ageing 25(8): 381–5.

Callum KG, Gray AJG, Vile RW, Ingram CS et al. (1999) Extremes of age. Report of the National Confidential Enquiry into Perioperative deaths. CEPOD, London.

Cameron I, Crotty M, Currie C, Finnegan T et al. (2000) Geriatric rehabilitation following fractures in older people: a systematic review. NHS R&D HTA Programme Health Technology Assessment 4(2).

Cameron ID, Alchin L, Cumming RG et al. (2002) Cognitive impairment, and dementia in frail older people predict falls: a prospective cohort study. International Symposium on Advances in Alzheimer Therapy, Geneva, 2002. www.siumed.educ/cme/12f.html.

Cameron ID, Handoll HHG, Finnegan TP, Madhok R et al. (2003) Co-ordinated multi-disciplinary approaches for in-patient rehabilitation of older patients with proximal femoral fractures. (Cochrane methodological review) Cochrane Library, Issue 4.

Campbell AJ, Robertson MC, Gardner MM et al. (1999) Falls prevention over two years. A randomised control trial in women over 80 years and older. Age and Ageing 28: 513–18.

Campbell D (2003) How acute renal failure puts the brakes on kidney function. Nursing 33(1): 59–63.

Campbell EM, Cater SE, Sanson-Fisher RW, Redman S et al. (1997) Environmental hazards in the homes of older people. Age and Ageing 26: 195–202.

Cannon CP, Hand MH, Bahr R et al. (2002) Critical pathways for management of patients with acute coronary syndromes: an assessment by the National Heart Attack Heart Plan. American Journal of Heart Surgery 143: 777–89.

Caress AL (2003) Giving information to patients. Nursing Standard 17(9): 45–50.

Casaletto J, Gatt R (2004) Post operative mortality related to waiting time for hip fracture surgery. Injury 35: 114–20.

Center JR, Nguynen TV, Pocock NA, Noakes KA et al. (1998) Femoral neck axis length, height loss and risk of hip fractures in males and females. Osteoporosis International 8: 75–81.

Chan DK, Hilier G, Loore M et al. (2000) Effectiveness and acceptability of a newly designed hip protector: a pilot study. Archives of Gerontology and Geriatrics 30: 25–34.

Chang ST, Morton SC, Rubenstein LZ et al. (2004) Interventions for the prevention of falls in older adults: systematic review and meta-analysis of randomised clinical trials. BMJ 328: 680.

Chapman A (1996) Current theory and practice: A study of pre-operative fasting. Nursing Standard 10(18): 33–6.

Chesser T, Howlett I, Ward A, Pounsford J (2002) The influence of outside temperature and season on the incidence of hip fractures in patients over the age of 65. Age and Ageing 31: 343–8.

Chilov MN, Cameron ID, March LM (2003) Evidence based guidelines for fixing broken hips. Cochrane Library, Issue 4.

Chin K, Evans MC, Cornish J, Cundy T et al. (1997) Differences in hip axis and femoral neck length in pre-menopausal women of Polynesian, Asian and European origin. Osteoporosis International 7: 344–7.

Chinoy MA, Parker MJ (1999) Fixed nail plates versus sliding hip systems for the treatment of trochanteric femoral fractures: a meta-analysis of 14 comparative studies. Injury 30(6): 157–63. (Erratum for Table 6, Injury 1999:30:452).

Chong PFM, Langerford AK, Dowsey MM, Santmaria NM (2000) Clinical pathway for fractured neck of femur: a prospective controlled study. Medical Journal of Australia 172: 423–6.

Clague JE, Craddock E, Andrew G, Horan MA, Pendleton P (2002) Predictors of out-come following hip fracture. Admission time predicts length of stay and in-hospital mortality. Injury 33(1): 1–6.

Clancy M, Roberts H (2000) Hip fractures: developing a break with tradition. Emergency Medicine 12: 274–5.

Clay M, Wade S (2003) Rehabilitation and older people. Nursing Older People 15(7): 25–9.

Clayer M, Brickner J (2000) Occult hypoxia after femoral neck fracture and elective hip surgery. Clinical Orthopedics 370: 265–71.

Clemson L, Cummings R, Roland M (1996) Case-control study of hazards and hip fracture. Ageing 25: 97–101.

Close J (2001) Interdisciplinary practice in the prevention of falls: a review of working models of care. Age and Ageing 30, suppl.4: 8–12.

Close J, Elis M, Hooper R et al. (1999) Prevention of falls in the elderly trial (PROFET): A randomised control trial. Lancet 353: 93–7.

Collins T (1999) Fractured neck of femur. Nursing Standard 13(23): 53–9.

Collins T (2000) Understanding shock. Nursing Standard 14(49): 35–9.

Compston JE (1994) Hormone replacement therapy for osteoporosis: clinical and pathophysiological aspects. Reproductive Medical Review 3: 209–24.

Compston JE, Rosen CR (1999) Osteoporosis, 2nd edn. Health Press, Oxford.

Connolly J, Cunningham AJ (2000) Pre-operative fasting and administration of regular medication in adult patients presenting for elective surgery. Has new evidence changed clinical practice? European Journal of Anaesthesiology 17: 219–20.

Cook MJ (1999) Improving care requires leadership in nursing. Nurse Education Today 19(4): 306–12.

Cooper AP (1822) A Treatise on Dislocations, and on Fractures of the Joints. Longman Hurst, Rees, Orme and Brown; E. Cox and Son. London. London.

Cooper C, Eriksson JG, Forsen T, Osmond C et al. (2001) Maternal height, childhood growth and risk of hip fracture in later life: a longitudinal study. Osteoprosis International 12: 623–9.

COP/BGS (2003) The importance of vision in preventing falls. College of Optometrists and British Geriatric Society, London.

Copeman J (1999) Nutritional Care for Older People. Age Concern, London.

Cree M, Carriere KC, Soskolne CL, Suarez-Almazor M (2001) Functional dependence after hip fracture. American Journal of Physical Medicine and Rehabilitation 80: 736–43.

CSP/COT (2000) The National Collaborative Audit for the Rehabilitative Management of Elderly People Who Have Fallen. Chartered Society of Physiotherapists and the College of Occupational Therapists, London.

Cullum N, Deeks JJ, Fletcher AW et al. (1995) Preventing and treating pressure sores. Quality in Health Care 4: 289–97.

Cumming RG, Klineber RJ (1993) Psychotropics, thiazide diuretics and hip fractures in the elderly. Medical Journal of Australia 158: 414–17.

Cumming RG, Thomas M, Szonyi G et al. (1999) Home visits by an occupational therapist for assessment and modification of environmental hazards: a randomised trial of falls prevention. Journal of the American Geriatric Society 47: 1379–1402.

Cummings S (1996) Treatable and untreatable risk factors for hip fracture. Bone 18: 165–167S.

Cummings SR, Browner WS, Bauer D, Stove K et al. (1998) Endogenous hormones and the risk of hip and vertebral fractures among older women. Study of Osteoporotic Fractures Research Group. New England Journal of Medicine 339: 733–8.

Cummings SR, Melton LJ (2002) Epidemiology and outcomes of osteoporotic fractures. Lancet 359(9319): 1761–1767.

Cunliffe A, Gladman, JRF, Husbands SL et al. (2004) Sooner and healthier: a randomised controlled trial and interview study of an elderly discharge rehabilitation services for older people. Age and Ageing 33: 246–252.

Cutfield G (2002) Anaesthesia and perioperative care for elderly surgical patients. Australian Prescriber 25: 42–44.

Dandy DJ, Edwards DJ (1998) Essential Orthopaedics and Trauma, 3rd edn. Churchill Livingstone, Edinburgh.

Darer J, Pronovost P, Bass EB (2002) Use and evaluation of critical pathways in hospitals. Effective Clinical Practice 5: 114–119.

Dargent-Molina P, Poitiers F, Breart G (2000) In elderly women weight is the best predictor of a very low bone mineral density: evidence from the EPIDOS study. Osteoporosis International 11: 881–888.

Davies C (2000) Getting health professionals to work together. BMJ 320: 1021–1022.

Davies C (2004) The use of phosphate enemas in the treatment of constipation. Nursing Times 100(18): 1–8.

Davies S (2001) The care needs of older people and family caregivers in continuing care settings. In: Nolan M et al. (eds) Working with Older People and Their Families. Open University Press, Buckingham.

De Jong MJ (1997) Clinical snapshot: cardiogenic shock. American Journal of Nursing 97(6): 40–41.

De Laine C, Scammell J, Heaslip V (2002) Continence care and policy initiatives. Nursing Standard 17(7): 45–51.

Delmas PD (2002) Treatment of post-menopausal osteoporosis. Lancet 359(9322): 2018–2026.

Dewing J (1999) Person centred dementia care: issues with theory and practice. Professional Nurse 14(9): 585–589.

Dewing J (2003) Rehabilitation for older people with dementia. Nursing Standard 18: 42–48.

Dey AB, Stout NR, Kenny RA (1997) Cardiovascular syncope is the most common cause of drop attacks in the elderly. Pacing Clinical Electrophysiology 20: 818–819.

DH (1995) Moving on: Report of the National Inspection of Social Services departments' arrangements for the discharge of older people from hospital to residential or nursing home care. Social Services Inspectorate, Department of Health. HMSO, London.

DH (1997) The new NHS: modern, dependable. Department of Health, London.

DH (1998a) A First Class Service: quality in the new NHS (White Paper). Department of Health, London.

DH (1998b) Clinical Governance: quality in the new NHS. Department of Health, London.

DH (1999) Making a Difference: strengthening the nursing, midwifery and health visiting contribution to health care. Department of Health, London.

DH (2000a) The NHS Plan: A plan for investment, A plan for reform. Department of Health, London.

DH (2000b) Survey of the NHS Infertility Services 1997–98. Department of Health, London.

DH (2000c) Good Practice in Continence Services. Department of Health, London.

DH (2001a) National Service Framework for Older People. Department of Health, London.

DH (2001b) Comprehensive Critical Care: a strategic programme of action. Department of Health, London.

DH (2001c) Guidance for Patient Consent. Department of Health, London.

DH (2001d) Seeking Consent: Working with Older People. Department of Health, London.

DH (2001e) NHS Funded Nursing Care – Practice Guide and Workbook. Department of Health, London.

DH (2001f) Building Capacity and Partnership in Care. Department of Health, London.

DH (2001g) Implementing the NHS Plan – Modern Matrons: Strengthening the role of ward sisters and introducing senior sisters. Health Service Circular 2001/010. Department of Health, London.

DH (2001h) Caring for Older People: A Nursing Priority. Integrating Knowledge, Practice and Values. Report by the Nursing and Midwifery Advisory Committee. Department of Health, London.

DH (2002a) Single Assessment Process. HSC 2002/001. Department of Health, London.

DH (2002b) Good Practice in Consent Implementation Guide: Consent to examination or treatment. Department of Health, London.

DH (2002c) Intermediate Care: moving forward. Department of Health, London.

DH (2002d) Modern Matrons in the NHS: A progress report. Department of Health, London.

DH (2002e) Care Homes for Older People and Younger Adults. National minimum standards for care homes for older people. National minimum standards for care homes for younger adults (18–65). Proposed amended environmental standards. Consultation document. Department of Health, London.

DH (2003a) Essence of Care: Patient-focused benchmarks for clinical governance. NHS Modernisation Agency, London.

DH (2003b) Critical Care Outreach: progress in developing services. Department of Health, London.

DH (2003c) Discharge from Hospital: pathway, process and practice. HMSO, London.

DH (2003d) Community Care (Delayed Discharges etc.) Act. The Stationery Office, London.

DH (2003e) Medical Stability and 'Safe to transfer'. Health and Social Care Change Agent Team/Reimbursement Implementation Team. Department of Health, London.

DH (2003f) Modern Matrons – improving the patient experience. Department of Health, London.

DH (2004) 4-Hour Checklist: reducing delays for A&E patients. Department of Health, London.

Dilsen G, Aydin R, Oral A, Sepici V et al. (1993) Regional differences in fracture risk in Turkey. Bone 14 (Suppl 1): 565–8.

Dinah AF (2003) Reduction of waiting times in A&E following introduction of 'fast track' scheme for elderly patients with a hip fracture. Injury 34: 839–41.

Dormenval V, Budtz-Jorgensen E, Mojon P et al. (1998) Association between malnutrition, poor general health and oral dryness in hospitalized elderly patients. Age and Ageing 27: 123–8.

DTB (1999) Drugs in the peri-operative period: 4 – Cardiovascular drugs. Drug and Therapeutic Bulletin 37(12): 89–92.

DTI (1999) Avoiding slips, trips and broken hips. Accidental falls in the home. Regional distribution of cases involving people aged over 65 in the UK. Department of Trade and Industry, London.

Eastell R, Reid DM, Compston J et al. (2001) Secondary prevention of osteoporosis: when should a non-vertebral fracture be a trigger for action? QJM 94: 575–97.

Easton KL (1999) Gerontological Rehabilitation Nursing. WB Saunders, London.

Eberhardie C (2003) Constipation. Identifying the problem. Nursing Older People 15(9): 22–6.

Edwards A (2002) A rehabilitation framework for patient focused care. Nursing Standard 16(50): 38–44.

Egol KA, Koval KJ (2002) Hip trauma. In: Koval KJ (ed.) Orthopaedic Knowledge Update 7. American Academy of Orthopaedic Surgeons, Rosemont, IL, pp 407–16.

Ellerby M (2003) Building a better future. In: Laings' Healthcare Market Review. Laing and Buisson, London.

Ellis J, Cooper A, Davis D et al. (2000) Making a difference to practice: clinical benchmarking part 2. Nursing Standard 14 (33): 32–5.

Ellis T (2003) Hip fractures in the elderly. Current Women's Health Reports 3: 75–80.

Evans EM (1949) The treatment of trochanteric fractures of the femur. Journal of Bone and Joint Surgery 31: 190–203.

Evans GJ, Tallis R (2001) A new beginning for care for elderly people. BMJ 322: 807–8.

Evans JR, Fletcher AE, Wormald RP et al. (2002) Prevalence of visual impairment in people aged 75 years and older in Britain: results from the MRC trial of assessment and management of older people in the community. British Journal of Ophthalmology 86: 795–800.

Everett B, Bridel-Nixon J (1997) The use of bed rails: principles of patient assessment. Nursing Standard 12(6): 44–7.

Fang MA, Frost PJ, Iida-Klein A, Hahn TJ (1991) Effects of nicotine on cellular function in UMR 106–01 osteoblast like cells. Bone 12: 283–6.

Feder G, Cryer C, Donovan S, Carter Y (2000) Guidelines for the prevention of falls in people over 65. BMJ 321(7267): 1007–11.

Fick D, Foreman M (2000) Consequences of not recognising delirium superimposed on dementia in hospitalized elderly individuals. Journal of Gerontological Nursing 26(1): 30–40.

Finch SA, Doyle W, Lowe CS et al. (1998) National Diet and Nutrition Survey: People Aged 65 and Over. Volume 1. Report of the diet and nutrition survey. The Stationery Office, London.

Fitzpatrick P, Kirke PN, Daly L, Van Rooij I et al. (2001) Predictors of first hip fracture and mortality post fracture in older women. Irish Journal of Medical Science 170(1): 49–53.

Folstein M, Folstein SE, McHugh PR (1975) Mini-mental state. A practical method for grading the cognitive state of patients for the clinician. Journal of Psychiatry and Research 12: 189–98.

Ford P, McCormack B (2000) Keeping the person in the centre of nursing. Nursing Standard 46(14): 40–4.

Forman H (1996) Relationship of malnutrition and length of stay in hospital. Journal of the American Dietetic Association 96 (Suppl): 29.

Forsen L, Bjartveit K, Bjorndal A, Edna TH et al. (1998) Ex-smokers and risk of hip fracture. American Journal of Public Health 88: 1481–3.

Fox KM, Cummings SR, Ponell-Threets K, Stone K (1998) Family history and risk of osteoporotic fracture. Study of osteoporotic research programme. Osteoporosis International 8(6): 557–62.

Frank PJ, Winterburg H, Moffatt C (1999) Quality of life in patients suffering from pressure ulceration: a case controlled study (Abstract). Ostomy and Wound Management 45: 56.

Freeman M, Miller C, Ross N (2000) The impact of individual philosophies of teamwork on multiprofessional practice and its implication for nursing. Journal of Interprofessional Care 46(14): 40–44.

Frels C, Williams P, Narayanan S, Gariballa SE (2002) Iatrogenic causes of falls in hospitalised elderly patients: a case control study. Postgraduate Medical Journal 78: 487–9.

Gaiballa SE, Sinclair AJ (1998) Nutrition, ageing and ill-health. British Journal of Nutrition 80: 7–23.

Garden RS (1961) Low angle fixation in fractures of the femoral neck. Journal of Bone and Joint Surgery 43: 647–63.

Gibson MJ, Andres RO, Isaacs B et al. (1987) The prevention of falls in later life. A report of the Kellogg International Group on the prevention of falls by the elderly. Danish Medical Bulletin 34(suppl. 4): 1–24.

Gilbert SS, Easy WR, Fitch WW (1995) The effect of pre-operative oral fluids on morbidity following anaesthetics for minor surgery. Anaesthesia 50(1): 79–81.

Gillespie LD, Gillespie WJ, Robertson MC et al. (2004) Interventions for preventing falls in elderly people (Cochrane review) Cochrane Library, Issue 1.

Gillespie WJ, Henry DA, O'Connell DL, Robertson J (2004) Vitamin D and vitamin D analogues for preventing fractures associated with involutional and postmenopausal osteoporosis (Cochrane review). Cochrane Library, Issue 2.

Gillespie WJ, Walenkamp G (2004) Antibiotic prophylaxis for surgery for proximal femoral and other closed long bone fractures (Cochrane review). Cochrane Library, Issue 2.

Gillick MR (2000) Rethinking the role of tube feeding in patients with advanced dementia. New England Journal of Medicine 342: 206–10.

GMC (2002) Withholding and Withdrawing Life Prolonging Treatment: Good Practice in Decision Making. General Medical Council, London.

Gnudi S, Ripamoriti C, Gualtieri G, Malavolta N (1999) Geometry of proximal femur in prediction of hip fracture in osteoporotic women. British Journal of Radiology 72(860): 729–33.

Goldacre M, Roberts S, Yeates D (2002) Mortality after admission to hospital with fractured neck of femur: database study. BMJ 325: 868–9.

Goldhill D, White S, Sumner A. (1999) Physiological values and procedures in the 24 hours before ICU admission from the ward. Anaesthesia 54: 529–34.

Goldstein FC, Strasser DC, Woodard JL, Roberts VJ (1997) Functional outcome of cognitively impaired hip fracture patients on a geriatric rehabilitation unit. Journal of the American Geriatric Society 45: 35–42.

Govier I (2000) Spiritual care in nursing; a systematic approach. Nursing Standard 14(17): 32–6.

Grant PT, Henry JM, McNaughton GW (2000) The management of elderly blunt trauma victims in Scotland: evidence of ageism. Injury 31: 519–29.

Gray CS, Gaskill D (1990) Cot sides. A continuing hazard for the elderly. Geriatric Medicine 20: 21–2.

Gregg EW, Pereira MA, Caspersen CJ (2000) Physical activity, falls and fractures among older adults: a review of the epidemiologic incidence. Journal of the American Geriatric Society 48(8): 883–93.

Grimes JP, Gregory PM, Noveck H et al. (2002) Time to surgery and mortality following hip fracture. American Journal of Medicine 112: 702–9.

Grisso JA, Chiu GY, Maislin G, Seinmann WC et al. (1991) Risk factors for hip fracture in men: a preliminary study. Journal of Bone and Mineral Research 6: 865–8.

Gunnes M, Mellstrom D, Johnell O (1998) How well can a previous fracture indicate a new fracture? A questionnaire study of 29,802 post-menopausal women. Acta Orthopaedica Scandinavica 69(5): 508–12.

HA/RCN (2000) Dignity on the Ward. Improving the experience of acute care for older people with dementia or confusion. A pocket guide for hospital staff. Help the Aged and the Royal College of Nursing, London.

Haddad FS, Williams RL, Prendergast CM (1996) The check X-ray: an unnecessary investigation after hip fracture fixation? Injury 27: 351–2.

Haines TP, Bennett KL, Osborne RH, Hill RD (2004) Effectiveness of targeted falls prevention programme in sub-acute hospital setting. Randomised controlled trial. BMJ 328: 726.

Hall SE, Williams JA, Senior JA, Goldswain PR et al. (2000) Hip fracture outcomes: quality of life and functional status in older adults living in the community. Australian and New Zealand Journal of Medicine 31: 327–32.

Hallier S, Cooper C, Kellingray S et al. (2000) Fluoride in drinking water and risk of hip fracture in the UK: A case control study. Lancet 355: 265–9.

Hancock S (2003) Intermediate care and older people. Nursing Standard 17(48): 45–51.

Handoll HHG, Farrar MJ, McBirnie J, Tytherleigh-Strong G et al. (2004) Heparin, low molecular weight heparin and physical methods for preventing deep vein thrombosis and pulmonary embolism following surgery for hip fractures (Cochrane review) Cochrane Lbrary, Issue 2.

Handoll HHG, Parker MJ, Sherrington C (2004) Mobilization strategies after hip fracture surgery in adults (Cochrane Review). Cochrane Library, Issue 1.

Hannan E, Magaziner J, Jason J, Wong E et al. (2001) Mortality and locomotion 6 months after hospitalization for hip fracture: risk factors and risk adjusted hospital outcomes. JAMA 285: 2736–42.

Harada A, Mizuno M, Takemura M et al. (2001) Hip fracture prevention trial using hip protectors in Japanese nursing homes. Osteoporosis International 12(3): 215–21.

Harvey I, Frankel S, Marks R et al. (1997) Foot morbidity and exposure to chiropody: population based study. BMJ 315: 1054–55.

HAS (1998/1999/2000) Not Because They Are Old – an independent enquiry into the care of older people on acute wards in general hospitals. Health Advisory Service, NHS Executive, London.

Hayes WC, Myers ER, Morris JN, Gerhart TN (1993) Impact near the hip dominates fracture risk in elderly nursing home residents who fall. Calcified Tissue International 52: 192–8.

HCA (2004) Protected Meal Times Policy. Hospital Caterers Association, London.

HCHC (2001) Delayed Discharges, Vol. 1. House of Commons Health Committee. The Stationery Office, London.

Healey F, Monro A, Cockram A, Adams V et al. (2004) Using targeted risk factor reduction to prevent falls in older in-patients: a randomised controlled trial. Age and Ageing 33: 390–5.

Healey WL, Iorio R, Ko J, Appleby D et al. (2002) Impact of cost reduction programmes on short term patient outcome and hospital costs of total knee arthroplasty. Journal of Bone and Joint Surgery 84A: 348–53.

Healthcare Commission (2004) Review of Implementation of the NSF for Older People. Healthcare Commission, London.

Heaton K (1999) Understanding Your Bowels. Family Doctor Publications, London.

Hefley FG, Nelson CL, Puskarich-May CL (1996) Effect of delayed admission to the hospital on the preoperative prevalence of deep vein thrombosis associated with fractures about the hip. Journal of Bone and Joint Surgery 78A: 581–3.

Heini P, Torsten F, Fankhauser C et al (2004) Femoroplasty-augmentation of mechanical properties in the osteoporotic proximal femur: a biomechanical investigation of PMMA reinforcement in cadaver bones. Clinical Biomechanics 19: 506–12.

Helford AE, Cook HL, Walinsky MD, Demp PH (1998) Foot problems associated with older patients a focused podogeriatric study. Journal of the American Podiatric Medical Association 88: 237–41.

Help the Aged (2000) Dignity on the Ward: promoting excellence in care, promoting practice in acute hospital care for older people. Help the Aged, London.

Help the Aged (2003) Falls Services. An overview of progress of falls prevention service developments against the milestones of the National Service Framework for Older People. Help the Aged, London.

Hemenway D, Azael DR, Rimm EB et al. (1994) Risk factors for hip fracture in US men aged 40 through 75 years. American Journal of Public Health 84(11): 1843–5.

Heruti RJ, Lusky A, Barell V, Adminsky A (1999) Cognitive status on admission: does it affect the rehabilitation outcomes of elderly patients with hip fracture? Archives of Physical Medicine and Rehabilitation 80: 432–6.

Hochberg M (2000) Preventing fractures in post-menopausal women with osteoporosis. A review of recent controlled trials of antiresorptive agents. Drugs and Ageing 17(4): 317–30.

Hodkinson HM (1972) Evaluation of a mental test score for assessment of mental impairment in the elderly. Age and Ageing 1(4): 233–8.

Hoidrup S, Prescott E, Sorensen T et al. (2000) Tobacco smoking and risk of hip fracture in men and women. International Journal of Epidemiology 29: P253–259.

Holmes S (2000) Nutritional screening and older adults. Nursing Standard 15(2): 42–4.

Holmes S (2003) Undernutrition in hospital patients. Nursing Standard 17(19): 45–52.

Holunberg-Martilla D, Sievanen H (1999) Prevalence of bone mineral change during post-partum amenrrhea and after resumption of menstruation. American Journal of Obstetrics and Gynaecology 180: 537–538.

Howell JM, Avolio B (1993) Transformational leadership, transactional leadership, locus of control and support for innovations: key predictors of consolidated business unit performance. Journal of Applied Psychology 78(6): 891–902.

Hughes A (2001) Recognising the causes of delirium in older people. Nursing Times 97(3). www.nursingtimes.net/nov?page=nt.print&resource213508.

Hung P (1992) Pre-operative fasting. Nursing Times 88: 57–60.

Huopio J, Kroger H, Honkenen R, Saarikoski S et al. (2000) Risk factors for perimenopausal fractures: a prospective stdy. Osteoporosis International 11: 219–27.

Huusko TM, Karppi P, Avikainen V, Kautiainen H et al. (2000) Randomised, clinically controlled trial of intensive geriatric rehabilitation in patients with hip fracture: subgroup analysis of patients with dementia. BMJ 321: 1107–11.

Ibbotson K (1999) The role of the clinical nurse specialist: a study. Nursing Standard 14(9): 45–48.

Ivers RQ, Cumming RG, Mitchell P et al. (1998) Visual impairment and falls in older people: The Blue Mountain eye study. Journal of the American Geriatric Society 46(1): 58–64.

Jacquim-Gadda H, Commenges D, Dartigues J-F (1995) Fluorine concentrations in drinking water and fractures in the elderly. JAMA 273: 775–6.

Jensen JS, Michaelson M (1975) Trochanteric femoral fractures treated with McLaughlin osteosynthesis. Acta Orthopaedica Scandinavica 46: 795–803.

Jester R, Williams S (1999) Pre-operative fasting: putting research into practice. Nursing Standard 13(39): 33–5.

Johnson S, Dracass BA, Varkin J, Eddington J (2000) Setting standards using Integrated Care Pathways. Professional Nurse 15(10): 640–3.

Jones G, Nguyen T, Sambrook PN, Eisman JA (1995) Thiazide diuretics and fractures: can meta-analysis help? Journal of Bone and Mineral Research 10: 106–11.

Jones H, Yates J, Spurgeon P, Fielder A (1996) Geographical variations in rates of ophthalmic surgery. British Journal of Ophthalmology 80: 784–8.

Juelsgaard P, Sand NP, Felsby S, Dalsgaard J et al. (1998) Perioperative myocardial ischaemia in patients undergoing surgery for fractured hip randomized to incremental spinal, single-dose spinal or general anaesthesia. European Journal of Anaesthesiology 15: 656–63.

Kamel HK, Phlavan M Malekgoudarzi B et al. (2001) Utilizing pain assessment scales increase the frequency of diagnosing pain among elderly nursing home residents. Journal of Pain and Symptom Management 21(6): 450–5.

Kanis JA, Johnell O, Oden A, Dawson A et al. (2001) Ten year probabilities of osteoporotic fractures according to BMD and diagnostic thresholds. Osteoporosis International 12: 989–95.

Karlsson KM, Sernbo I, Obrant KJ, Redland-Johnell I et al. (1996) Femoral neck geometry and radiographic signs of osteoporosis as predictors of hip fracture. Bone 18: 327–30.

Keady J, Bender MP (1998) Changing faces: the purpose and practice of assessing older adults with cognitive impairment. Health Care in Later Life 3(2): 129–43.

Kelly A, Dowling M (2004) Reducing the likelihood of falls in older people. Nursing Standard 15(49): 33–40.

Kelly KD, Malone B, Hempel P, Voaklander D (2000) Orthopaedic subacute rehabilitation – predictors of functional outcome and resource utilization. International Journal of Rehabilitation and Health 5(3): 165–76.

Kenny G (2002) Interprofessional working: opportunities and challenges. Nursing Standard 17(6): 33–5.

Kenny RA, Richardson DA, Steen IN (2001) Carotid sinus syndrome is modifiable risk factor for nonaccidental falls in older adults. Journal of the American College of Cardiology 38(5): 1491–6.

Kitwood A (1997) Dementia Reconsidered. The person comes first. Open University Press, Buckingham.

Kramer A, Angst M, Gasser B, Ganz R (2000) [Increasing bone screw anchoring in the femur head by cement administration via the implant – a biomechanical study]. Zeitschrift für Orthopädie und ihre Grenzgebiete 5: 464–9 (in German).

Kujala VM, Kaprio J, Kannus P, Sarvna S et al. (2000) Physical activity and osteoporotic hip fracture risk in men. Archives of Internal Medicine 160(5) 705–8.

Kumar NP, Thomas A, Mudd P et al. (2003) The usefulness of carotid sinus massage in different patient groups. Age and Ageing 32: 666–9.

Kwan J, Sandercock P (2002) In-hospital care pathways for stroke (Cochrane review). Cochrane Database Systemic Review 2:CD002924.

Kwong L (2003) Balancing new technology with established techniques. www.orthobluejournal.com/suppl0803/kwong.asp

Lane NE (2001) An update on glucocorticoid-induced osteoporosis. Rheumatological Disease Clinics of North America 27(1): 235–53.

Larsson S, Bauer TW (2002) Use of injectable calcium phosphate cement for fracture fixation: a review. Clinical Orthopedics 395: 23–32.

Lau EM, Lee JK, Suriwongpaisal P, Saw SM et al. (2001) The incidence of hip fracture in four Asian countries: the Asian Osteoporosis Study (AOS). Osteoporosis International 12(3): 239–43.

Law G (2003) Developing the nurse's role in rehabilitation. Nursing Standard 17(45): 33–8.

Laxton C, Freeman C, Todd C, Payne B et al. (1997) Morbidity at three months after hip fracture: data from the East Anglian Audit. Health Trends 29: 55–60.

Lieberman D, Fied V, Castel H, Weitzmann S et al. (1996) Factors related to successful rehabilitation after hip fracture: a case control study. Disability Rehabilitation 5: 224–30.

Lord S, Sherrington C, Menz H (2001) Falls in Older People. Risk Factors and Strategies for Prevention. Cambridge University Press, Cambridge.

Lord SR, Bashford GM (1996) Shoe characteristics and balance in older women. Journal of the American Geriatric Society 44(4): 429–33.

Luker KA, Waters KR (1996) Staff perspectives of the role of the nurse in rehabilitation wards for the elderly. Journal of Clinical Nursing 5: 105–14.

Lunsjo K, Ceder L, Thorngren KG, Skytting B et al. (2001) Extramedullary fixation of 569 unstable trochanteric fractures: a randomized multicenter trial of the Medoff sliding plate versus three other screw-plate systems. Acta Orthopaedica Scandinavica 72(2): 133–40.

Luthje P, Peltonen A, Nurmi I, Kataja M et al. (1995) No differences in incidence of old people's hip fracture between urban and rural populations – a comparative study in two Finnish health care regions in 1989. Gerontology 41(1): 39–44.

Luukinen H, Koski K, Kivela SL, Laippala P (1996) Social status, life changes, housing conditions, health, functional abilities and life-style as risk factors for recurrent falls among the home dwelling elderly. Public Health 110: 115–18.

Lyons ARC (1997) Clinical outcomes and treatment of hip fracture. American Journal of Medicine 103: 51–64.

Macintyre P, Ready L (2001) The DOLOPLUS 2 Scale- evaluating pain in the elderly. European Journal of Palliative Care 8(5): 191–4.

Madhok R, Melton LJ III, Atkinson EJ, O'Fallan WM et al (1993) Urban versus rural increase in hip fracture incidence. Age and sex of 907 cases 1980–89 in Olmsted County USA. Acta Orthopaedica Scandinavica 64(5): 543–8.

Magaziner J, Hawkes W, Hebel J, Zimmerman I (2000) Recovery from hip fracture in eight areas of function. Journals of Gerontology A 55: M498–M507.

Mahoney FI, Barthel DW (1965) Functional evaluation: The Barthel Index. Maryland State Medical Journal 14: 61–5.

Mahoney JE (1998) Immobility and falls. Clinical Geriatric Medicine 14: 99–227.

Malone-Lee J (2000) The elderly. In: Stanton SL, Merga AK (eds). Clinical Gynaecology. Churchill Livingstone, London.

Manley K (1997) A conceptual framework for advanced practice: an action research project operationalizing an advanced practitioner/consultant nurse role. Journal of Clinical Nursing 6: 179–90.

Manyon-Davis A, Bristow A (1999) Managing Nutrition in Hospital: a recipe for quality. Nuffield Trust, London.

Marcantonio ER, Flacker JM, Michaels M, Resnick NM (2000) Delirium is an independently associated with poor functional recovery after hip fracture. Journal of the American Geriatric Society 48(6): 618–24.

Marks R (1996) Practical Problems in Dermatology. Chapman & Hall, London.

Marsh D (2003) Burning issues in fracture science management. The Robert Jones Lecture, presented at the British Orthopaedic Association annual conference, September 17–19, 2003. Birmingham. England. Quoted in Orthopaedics Today International Jan/Feb 2004, p.10.

Marshall Z, Luffingham P (1998) Does the specialist nurse enhance or deskill the general nurse? British Journal of Nursing 1998 7(11): 658–62.

Martin C (2000) A pressure damage prevention strategy. NT plus (with Nursing Times) 96(36).

McArthur-Rouse F (2001) Critical care outreach services and early warning scoring systems; a review of the literature. Journal of Advanced Nursing 36(5): 696–704.

McCormack B (1999) The contribution of expert gerontological nursing. Nursing Standard 13(25): 42–5.

McCormack B (2001) Clinical effectiveness and clinical teams: effective practice with older people. Nursing Older People 13(5): 14–17.

McCosty DJ, Coopman WJ (1993) Osteoporotic bone diseases. In: Berra et al. (eds) Arthritis and Allied Conditions – a textbook of rheumatology. Lea and Febinger, Philadelphia.

McCrae R (1983) Practical Fracture Treatment. Churchill Livingstone, Edinburgh.

McCreadie M (2001) The role of the clinical nurse specialist. Nursing Standard 16(10): 33–8.

McGough AJ (1999) A systematic review of the effectiveness of risk assessment scales used in the prevention and management of pressure sores. MSc. Thesis, University of York.

McGrother CW, Donaldson MM, Clayton D, Abrams KR, Clarke M (2002) Evaluation of a hip fracture risk score for assessing elderly women: the Melton Osteoporotic Fracture (MOF) study. Osteoporosis International 13: 89–96.

McMurdo MET, Millar AM, Daly F (2000) A randomized controlled trial of fall prevention strategies in old peoples' homes. Gerontology 46(2): 83–7.

McWilliams CL, Wong CA (1994) Keeping it secret: the costs and benefits of nursing's hidden work in discharging patients. Journal of Advanced Nursing 19: 152–63.

Melton LJ 3rd (1993) Hip fractures: a worldwide problem today and tomorrow. Bone 14 Suppl 1: S1–8.

Menz HB, Lord SR (2001) Foot pain impairs balance and functional ability in community dwelling older people. Journal of the American Podiatric Medical Association 91(5): 222–9.

Meyer G, Warnke A, Bender R et al. (2003) Effect on hip fracture of increased use of hip protectors in nursing homes: cluster randomized controlled trial. BMJ 326: 76–81.

Michaelson K, Baron JA, Faralmond BY, Ljunghall S (2001) Influence of parity and lactation on hip fracture risk. American Journal of Epidemiology 153: 1166–72.

Michelloti J, Clark J (1999) Femoral neck length and hip fracture risk. Journal of Bone and Mineral Research 14: 1714–20.

Middleton S, Roberts A, Reeves D (2000) What is an ICP? www.evidence-based-medicine.co.uk.

Miller L (2002) Effective communication with older people. Nursing Standard 17(9): 45–50.

Milne AC, Potter J, Avenell A (2004) Protein and energy supplementation in elderly people at risk from malnutrition. (Cochrane Review). Cochrane Library, Issue 2.

Mitchell S, Berekowitz RE, Lawson FME, Lipsitz LA (2000) A cross national survey of tube feeding decisions in cognitively impaired older persons. Journal of the American Geriatric Society 48: 391–7.

Mohanty K, Gupta SK, Evans RM (2000) Check radiography after fixation of hip fractures: is it necessary? Journal of the Royal College of Surgeons of Edinburgh 45: 398–9.

Morrison R, Siu A (2000) A comparison of pain and its treatment in advanced dementia and cognitively intact patients with hip fracture. Journal of Pain and Symptom Management 19(4): 240–8.

Morrison RS, Magaziner J, Gilbert M, Koval KJ et al. (2003) Relationship between pain and opioid analgesics in the development of delirium following hip fracture. Journal of Gerontology A 58(1): 76–81.

Mow VA, Hayes WC (1997) Basic Orthopaedic Biomechanics, 2nd edn. Lippincott Williams & Wilkins, New York.

Mulholland H (2003) Sloppy slippers scheme cuts older peoples falls. Guardian, Tuesday 23 December. society.guardian.co.uk/longtermcare/story Mulron CD, Geretym B, Kauten D et al. (1994) Physical rehabilitation for very frail nursing home residents. JAMA 271: 519–24.

Murphy SL, Dubin J, Thomas G (2003) The development of fear of falling among community living older women: predisposing factors and subsequent fall events. Journal of Gerontology A 58: M943–M947.

Nakamura T, Turner CH, Yoshikawa T, Slemenda CW et al. (1994) Do variations in hip geometry explain differences in hip fracture risk between Japanese and White Americans? Journal of Bone and Mineral Research 9: 1071–6.

National Audit Office (2003) Ensuring the Effective Discharge of Older Patients from NHS Acute Hospitals. Report by the Comptroller and Auditor General. National Audit Office, London.

National Osteoporosis Society (2001) Position statement on the use of peripheral x-ray asorptiometry in the management of Osteoporosis. National Osteoporosis Society, London.

NCEPOD (1999) Extremes of Age. Report of the National Confidential Enquiry into Patient Outcome and Death. National Confidential Enquiry into Perioperative Deaths, London.

Netten A, Darton R, Williams J (2003) Nursing home closures: effects on capacity and reason for closure. Age and Ageing 32: 332–7.

Nevitt MC, Moss PD, Pamermo L, Musliner T et al. (1999) Association of prevalent vertebral fractures, bone density and alendronate treatment with incident vertebral fractures: effect of number and spinal location of fractures. The Fracture Intervention Trial Research Group. Bone 25(5): 613–19.

New Generation Project (2003) www.mhbs.soton.ac.uk/newgeneration.

Newkirk MR Van, Weih L, McCarty CA, Taylor HR (2001) Case specific prevalence of bilateral visual impairment in Victoria, Australia – The visual improvement project. Ophthalmology 108(5): 960–7.

NHSE (1999) Nurse, midwife and health visitor consultants – establishing posts and making appointments. Health Service Circular 217, NHS Executive, London.

NICE (2001a) Inherited clinical guidelines B. Pressure ulcer risk assessment and prevention. National Institute for Clinical Excellence, London.

NICE (2001b). Guidance on the use of cyclo-oxygenase (COX) II selective inhibitors, celexcoxib, rafecoxib, meloxicam and etodalac for Osteoarthritis and Rheumatoid Arthritis. National Institute for Clinical Excellence, London.

NICE (2004) Falls. The assessment and prevention of falls in older people. National Institute for Clinical Excellence, London.

Nicklin J (2002) Improving the quality of written information for patients. Nursing Standard 16(49): 39–44.

Nightingale S, Holmes J et al. (2001) Psychiatric illness and mortality after hip fracture. Lancet 357: 1264–5.

Nolan M (2000) Skills for the future: the humanity of caring. Nursing Management 7(6): 22–9.

Normann HK, Asplund K, Norberg A (1999) Attitudes of registered nurses towards patients with severe dementia. Journal of Clinical Nursing 8(4): 353–9.

Norton D (1989) Calculating the risk: reflections on the Norton scale. Decubitus 2(3): 24–31.

Notre Dame (2002) Quality of life: the next frontier for engineers. www.nd.edu/engineer/publications/signatures/2002/biomechanic/html.

O'Halloran D, Cran G, Beringer T et al (2004) A cluster randomized controlled trial to evaluate a policy of making hip protectors available to residents of nursing homes. Age and Ageing 33: 582–8.

O'Toole GC (2002) Hip protectors and the elderly. Irish Medical Journal 95(6): 165.

Oliver D (2004) Prevention of falls in hospital in-patients. Agendas for research and practice. Age and Ageing 33: 328–30.

Oliver D, Brittan M, Seed P, Martin P et al. (1997) Development and evaluation of an evidence based risk assessment tool (STRATIFY) to predict which elderly inpatients will fall: case control and cohort studies. BMJ 315: 1049–53.

Oliver D, Daly F, Marion E, McMurdo T (2004) Risk factors and risk assessment tools for falls in hospital in-patients: a systematic review. Age and Ageing 33: 122–30.

Onslow E, Roberts H, Steiner A, Powell J, Pickering RM (2003) An integrated care pathway for fractured neck of femur patients. Professional Nurse 18: 265–8.

Ooms ME, Lips P, Van Lingen A, Valkenburg HA (1993) Determinants of bone mineral density and risk factors for osteoporosis in healthy elderly women. Journal of Bone and Mineral Research 8: 669–75.

Packwood T, Kober A (1995) Clinical Audit and its relationship to other forms of quality assurance and knowledge generation. In: Kogan M, Redfern S (eds) Making Use of Clinical Audit: a guide to practice in the health professions. Open University Press, Buckingham.

Paillaud E, Merlier I, Dupeyron C et al. (2004). Oral candidiasis and nutritional deficiencies in elderly hospitalised patients. British Journal of Nutrition 92(5) 861–7.

Paley G (1995) A framework for clinical protocols. Nursing Standard 9(21): 33–5.

Parker MJ, Currie TC, Morton JA, Therngren KG (1998) Standardised audit of hip fracture in Europe (SAHFE). Hip International 8: 10–15.

Parker MJ, Gillespie LD, Gillespie WJ (2005) Hip protectors for preventing hip fractures in the elderly. (Cochrane review). Cochrane Library, Issue 1.

Parker MJ, Gursamy K (2004) Arthroplasties (with and without bone cement) for proximal femoral fractures in adults. Cochrane Library, Issue 2.

Parker MJ, Handoll HH, Bhagara A (2004) Conservative versus operative treatment for hip fractures (Cochrane review). Cochrane Library, Issue 2.

Parker MJ, Handoll HHG (2003a) Gamma and other cephalcondylic intramedullary nail versus extramedullary implants for extracapsular hip fractures (Cochrane review). Cochrane Library, Issue 1.

Parker MJ, Handoll HHG (2003b) Extramedullary fixation implants and external fixators for extracapsular hip fractures (Cochrane review). Cochrane Library, Issue 1.

Parker MJ, Handoll HHG, Griffiths R, Unwin SC (2004) Anaesthesia for hip fracture surgery in adults (Cochrane review). Cochrane Library, Issue 2.

Parker MJ, Palmer CR (1995) Prediction of rehabilitation after hip fracture. Age and Ageing 24: 496–8.

Parker MJ, Pryor GA (1993) Handbook of Hip Fracture Surgery. Blackwell Scientific Publications, Oxford.

Parker MJ, Roberts C (2004) Closed suction surgical wound drainage after Orthopaedic Surgery. (Cochrane Review). Cochrane Library, Issue 2.

Parker MJ, Stockton G (2003) Internal fixation implants for intracapsular proximal femoral fractures in adults (Cochrane review). Cochrane Library, Issue 1.

Parker MJ, Tagg CE (2002) Internal fixation of intracapsular fractures. Journal of the Royal College of Surgeons of Edinburgh 47(3): 541–7.

Parker MJ, Tivemlow TR, Pryor GA (1996) Environmental hazards and hip fractures. Age and Ageing 25(4): 322–5.

Pasero C, Reed BA, McCaffery M (1999) Pain in the elderly. In: McCaffrey M, Pasero C (eds.) Pain: clinical manual, 2nd edn. Mosby, St. Louis, Mo.

Payne S, Kerr C, Hawker S, Hardy M et al. (2002) The communication of information about older people between health and social care practitioners. Age and Ageing 31: 107–17.

Pearse R, Rajakulendran (1999) Pre-operative fasting and administration of regular medications in adult patients presenting for elective surgery. Has the new evidence changed practice? European Journal of Anaesthesiology 16: 565–8.

PEP Trial (2000) Prevention of pulmonary embolism and deep vein thrombosis with low dose aspirin: Pulmonary Embolism Prevention (PEP) Trial. Lancet 355 (9212): 1295–302.

Perdue C (2003) Falls in older people; taking a multidisciplinary approach. Nursing Times 99(31): 1–6.

Petterson T (1994) How readable are the hospital information leaflets available to the elderly? Age and Ageing 23(1): 14–16.

Phillips S, Hutchinson S, Davidson T (1993) Preoperative drinking does not effect gastric contents. British Journal of Anaesthesia 70(1): 6–9.

Phipps K, Orwell E, Mason J, Cauley J (2000) Community water fluoridation, bone mineral density and fractures – prospective study of effects in older women. BMJ 321: 860–4.

PSSRU (2003) Cognitive Impairment in Older People: its implications for future demand for services. LSE Health and Social Care Discussion Paper 1728.

Quereshi A, Seymour DG (2003) Growing knowledge about hip fracture in older people. Age and Ageing 32: 8–9.

Rajmohan B (2000) Audit of the effect of a fast tracking protocol on transfer time from A&E to ward for patients with hip fractures. Injury 33(1): 1–6.

RCN (1999) Royal College of Nursing Ward Leadership Programme. Royal College of Nursing, London.

RCN (2000) Rehabilitation: The role of the nurse. Workbook. Royal College of Nursing, London.

RCN (2001) Clinical Practice Guidelines: Pressure ulcer risk assessment and prevention recommendations. Royal College of Nursing, London.

RCN (2004) Digital Rectal Examination and Manual Removal of Faeces. Royal College of Nursing, London.

RCP (1989) Fractured neck of femur. Prevention and management. Summary and recommendations of a report of the Royal College of Physicians. Journal of the Royal College of Physicians. 23: 8–12.

RCP (1999) Osteoporosis – clinical guidelines for prevention and treatment. Royal College of Physicians, London.

RCP (2002) Nutrition and Patients: a doctor's responsibility. Royal College of Physicians, London.

RCP (2003) Myocardial Infarction National Audit Project report. April 2002–March 2003. Clinical effectiveness and evaluation unit. Royal College of Physicians, London.

RCP (2004) National Sentinel Stroke Audit. Prepared on behalf of the Intercollegiate Stroke Working Party. Clinical Effectiveness and Evaluation Unit. Royal College of Physicians, London.

RCP/BTS (1999) Osteoporosis. Clinical guidelines for prevention and treatment. Royal College of Physicians/Bone and Tooth Society, London.

RCP/BTS/NOP (2002) Glucocorticoid-induced osteoporosis. Guidelines for prevention and treatment. Royal College of Physicians/Bone and Tooth Society of Great Britain/National Osteoporosis Society, London.

Redfern L (2003) Clinical pinnacle. Nursing Standard 17(22): 96.

Redmond S, McDevitt M, Barnes S (2004) Acute renal failure: recognition and treatment in ward patients. Nursing Standard 18(22): 46–53.

Richardson DA, Bexton RS, Shaw FE et al. (1997) Prevalence of cardioinhibitory carotid sinus hypersensitivity in patients 50 years or over presenting in the Accident and Emergency Department with unexplained or recurrent falls. Pacing and Clinical Electrophysiology 20: 820–3.

Richmond J (2003) Prevention of constipation through risk management. Nursing Standard 17(16): 39–46.

Richmond J, Ahraonoff GB, Zuckerman JD, Koval KJ (2003) Mortality risk after hip fracture. Journal of Orthopedic Trauma 17(1): 53–6.

Richy F, Bousquet J, Ehrlich GE, Meunier PJ et al. (2003) Inhaled corticosteroids effects on bone in asthmatic and COPD patients: a quantitative systematic review. Osteoporosis International 14: 179–90.

Robbins S, Waked E, Allard P et al. (1997) Foot position awareness in younger and older men: the influence of footwear sole properties. Journal of the American Geriatric Society 45: 61–6.

Roberts H, Pickering R, Onslow E, Clancy M et al. (2004) The effectiveness of implementing a care pathway for femoral neck fracture in older people: a prospective controlled before and after study. Age and Ageing 33: 178–84.

Roberts H, Steiner A, Powell J, Onslow E et al. (2002) The hidden costs of implementing a care pathway. Age and Ageing 31: 47.

Robertson MC, Devlin N, Schuffhan P et al (2001) Economic evaluation of a community based exercise programme to prevent falls. Journal of Epidemiology and Community Health 55: 600–6.

Robinson SB (1999) Transitions in the lives of elderly women who have sustained hip fractures. Journal of Advanced Nursing 30: 1341–8.

Röder F, Schwab M, Aleker T et al. (2003) Proximal femur fracture in older patients – rehabilitation and clinical outcome Age and Ageing 32: 74–80.

Rodgers S (2000) The patient facing surgery. In: Alexander M et al. (eds). Nursing Practice: hospital and home. The Adult. London. Churchill Livingstone, Edinburgh.

Rodriguez C (2001) Pain measurement in the elderly: a review. Pain Management Nursing 2(2): 38–46.

Roe B, Webb C (1998) Research and Development in Clinical Nursing Practice. Whurr Publishers, London.

Rosell PA, Parker MJ (2003) Functional outcomes after hip fracture. A 1-year prospective outcome study of 275 patients. Injury 34(7): 529–32.

Rosenberg J, Penderson MH, Gebuhr P, Kehler H (1992) Effects of oxygen therapy on late postoperative episodic and constant hypoxaemia. British Journal of Anaesthesia 68: 18–22.

Rothera I, Jones RG, Harwood RH, Waite J et al. (2003) Health status and assessed need for a cohort of older people admitted to nursing and residential homes. Age and Ageing 32: 303–9.

Rubenstein LZ, Josephson KR, Trueblood PR et al. (2000) Effects of a group exercise programme on strength, mobility and falls among fall prone elderly men. Journal of Gerontology A 55: M317–M321.

Rudberg MA, Egleston BL, Grant MD, Brody JA (2000) Effectiveness of feeding tubes in nursing home residents with swallowing disorders. JPEN 24: 97–102.

Rutledge D, Donaldson N (1998) Pain assessment and documentation, Part 1. Overview and application in adults. Online Journal of Clinical Innovations 1. www.cinahl. com/cgi-bin/ojcishowdoc3.cgi?vol01.htm.

Ryan J (1999) Communication with older people. In: Arnold E, Underman Boggs K (eds) Interpersonal Relationships: Professional communication skills for nursing, 3rd edn. WB Saunders, Philadelphia, PA.

Ryan N (1996) The right track. Nursing Times 41: 92.

Salgado R, Lord SR, Packer J, Ehrlich F (1994) Factors associated with falling in elderly hospital patients. Gerontology 40: 325–31.

Salkeld G, Cameron ID, Cumming RG, Easter S et al. (2000) Quality of life related to fear of falling and hip fracture in older women: a time trade off study. BMJ 320: 341–6.

Salmon D, Jones M (2001) Shaping the interprofessional agenda: a study examining qualified nurses perception of working with others. Nurse Education Today 21(1): 18–25.

Sander R (2002) Rehabilitation in the community. Nursing Older People 14(3): 10–13.

Sashkin M, Rosenbach WE (1993) A new leadership paradigm. In: Rosenbach WE, Taylor RL (eds) Contemporary Issues in Leadership, 3rd edn. Westview Press, Boulder, CO, pp 87–108.

Sattin RW, Rodriguez JG, DeVito CA et al. (1998) Home environmental hazards and the risk of falls injury events among community dwelling older persons. Study to assess falls among the elderly (SAFE) group. Journal of the American Geriatric Society 46: 669–76.

Schofield I, Dewing J (2001) The nursing contribution to the care of older people with a delirium in acute care settings. Nursing Older People 13(1): 21–5.

Schweitzer A (1953) On the Edge of the Primeval Forest. Adam and Charles Black, London.

Scottish Hip Fracture Audit Report (2002) Scottish Hip Fracture Audit Report. Scottish Office and NHS Executive, Edinburgh.

Scottish Office (1993) Clinical resources and audit group clinical guidelines: report by a working group. Scottish Office, Edinburgh.

Scott-Russell A, Dennison E, Cooper C (2003). Epidemiology and public health impact of osteoporosis. Chapter 2 in New A, Bonjour J-P (eds) Nutritional Aspects of Bone Health. Royal Society of Chemistry, Cambridge.

Scriven A, Tucker C (1997) The quality and management of written information presented to women undergoing hysterectomy. Journal of Clinical Nursing 6(2): 107–13.

Seedhouse DF (1998) The Heart of Health Care. John Wiley & Sons, Chichester.

Seinheimer F (1978) Subtrochanteric fractures of the femur. Journal of Bone and Joint Surgery 60A: 300–6.

Shah MR, Aharonoff G, Wollinsky P (2001) Outcomes after hip fracture in individuals ninety years of age and older. Journal of Orthopedic Trauma 15: 34–9.

Sharrock NE (2000) Fractured neck of femur in the elderly. Intensive perioperative care is warranted. British Journal of Anaesthesia 84: 139–40.

Shaw F, Bond J, Richardson D et al. (2003) Multifactorial interventions after a fall in older people with cognitive impairment and dementia presenting to the Accident and Emergency Department: A randomised control trial. BMJ 326: 73.

Shaw F, Kenny R (1998) Can falls in patients with dementia be prevented? Age and Ageing 27(1):7–9.

Sheehan J, Mohamed F, Reilly M, Perry IJ. (2000) Secondary prevention following fractured neck of femur: a survey of orthopaedic surgeons practice. Irish Medical Journal 93:105–107.

SIGN (2002) Guideline 56. Prevention and management of hip fracture in older people. Scottish Intercollegiate Guidelines Network. www.sign.ac.uk/guidelines/fulltext/56.

Silk D, Menzies Gow N (2001) Post-operative starvation after gastrointestinal surgery. BMJ 323(736): 761–2.

Smeeth L, Illiffe S (1998) Effectiveness of screening older people for impaired vision in community settings: systemic review of evidence from randomised control trials. BMJ 316: 660–3.

Smeltzer S, Bare B (2000) Brunner and Sudarth's Textbook of Medical-Surgical Nursing, 9th edn. Lippincott, Philadelphia, PA.

Smith G (2000) ALERT: Acute Life Threatening Events Recognition and Treatment. University of Portsmouth, Portsmouth.

Smith S (2000) Catch all solution. Nursing Times 96 (3): 22–3.

Smoker A (1999) Skin care in old age. Nursing Standard 13(48): 47–53.

Sowers M (1996) Pregnancy and lactation as risk factors for subsequent bone loss and osteoporosis. Journal of Bone and Mineral Research 11: 1052–60.

Steiner JF, Kramer AM, Eilertsen TB, Kowalsky JC (1997) Development and validation of a clinical prediction rule for prolonged nursing home residence after hip fracture. Journal of the American Geriatric Society 45(12): 1510–14.

Stevenson B, Mills EM, Welin L, Beal KG (1998) Falls risk factors in an acute care setting: a retrospective study. Canadian Journal of Nursing Research 30: 97–111.

Stevenson J (1999) Comprehensive Assessment of Older People: King's Fund Rehabilitation Programme. Developing rehabilitation opportunities for older people. King's Fund, London.

Stevenson J, Spencer L (2002) Developing Intermediate Care: A guide for health and social services professionals. King's Fund, London.

Stokes G (2000) Challenging Behaviour in Dementia: a person centred approach. Winslow, Bicester.

Stratton RJ, Hackston A, Longmore D et al. (2004) Malnutrition in hospital outpatients and in patients: prevalence, concurrent validity, and ease of use of the 'Malnutrition Universal Screening Tool' ('MUST') for adults. British Journal of Nutrition 92: 799–808.

Sulch D, Evans A, Melbourn A, Kalra L (2002) Does an integrated care pathway improve processes of care in stroke rehabilitation? A randomized control trial. Age and Ageing 31: 175–9.

Sulch D, Perez I, Melbourn A, Kalra L (2000) Evaluation of an integrated care pathway for stroke unit rehabilitation. Age and Ageing 29: 87.

Sullivan R, Badros K(1999) Recognize risk factors to prevent patient falls. Nursing Management 30(5): 37–40.

Sutherland S (1999) With Respect to Old Age: Long term care, rights and responsibilities. A report by the Royal Commission on Long Term Care. The Stationery Office, London.

Sweeney AB, Flora HS, Chaloner EJ, Buckland J et al. (2002) Integrated care pathways for vascular surgery: an analysis of the first 18 months. Postgraduate Medical Journal 78: 175–7.

Taraborrelli P, Wood F, Bloor M, Pithouse A et al. (1998) Hospital discharge for frail older people. Central Research Unit, Scottish Office, Edinburgh.

Tavener T (2002) Elderly care nurses' knowledge. Nursing Times 98(32). 1 5.

Theobold TM, Cauley JA, Gluer CC, Bunke CH et al. (1998) Black-white differences in hip geometry. Study of the Osteoprosis Fractures Research Group. Osteoporosis International 8(1): 61–67.

Thorkildsen K (2000) Patients with hip fracture – their experiences from the preoperative period. www.uib.no/isf/people/doc/hovedfag/nursing/karimt.htm.

Tiiana H, Pertti K, Veukko A, Hannu K et al. (2000) 2000). Randomised, clinically controlled trial of intensive geriatric rehabilitation in patients with hip fracture; sub group analysis of patients with dementia. BMJ 321: 1107–11.

Tinnetti ME, Inouye SK, Gill TM, Doucette JT (1995) Shared risk factors for falls, incontinence, and functional dependence. Unifying the approach to geriatric syndromes. JAMA 273: 1348–1353.

Todd CJ, Freeman CT, Camilleri-Ferrante C, Palmer CR et al. (1995) Differences in mortality after fractures of the hip: The East Anglian Audit. BMJ 310: 904–8.

Torgerson D, Inglesias C, Reid D (2000) The economics of fracture prevention. NOS press release, 8 December.

Torgerson DJ, Dolan P (1998) The cost of treating osteoporotic fractures in the UK female population. Osteoporosis International 8: 611–17.

Torgerson DJ, Iglesias CP, Reid DM (2001) The economics of fracture prevention. In: Barlow DH (ed) The Effective Management of Osteoporosis. Aesculapius Medical Press, London, pp. 111–21.

Tromp AM, Ooms ME, Popp-Snijders E et al. (2000). Predictors of fractures in elderly women. Osteoporosis International 11: 134–40.

US Congress (1994) Hip Fracture outcomes in people aged 50 and over. Office of Technology Assessment Background Paper OTA-BP-H-120. US Government Printing Office, Washington, DC.

van der Pols JC, Bates CJ, McGraw PV et al. (2000) Visual acuity measurements in a national sample of British elderly people. British Journal of Ophthalmology 84: 165–170.

van Doorn C, Gruber-Baldini A, Zimmerman S, Habel J et al. (2003) Dementia as a risk factor for falls and falls injuries among nursing home residents (abstract). Journal of the American Geriatric Society 51(9): 1213.

van Newkirk MR, Weih L, McCarty CA, Taylor HR (2001) Case specific prevalence of bilateral visual impairment in Victoria, Australia – the visual improvement project. Ophthalmology 108(5): 960–7.

van Staa TP, Denison EM, Leufkens HGM, Cooper C (2001) Epidemiology of fractures in England and Wales. Bone 29: 517–22.

van Staa TP, Leufkens HGM, Cooper C (2002a) The epidemiology of corticosteroidinduced osteoporosis: a meta-analysis. Osteoporosis International 13: 777–87.

Van Staa TP, Leufkens HG, Cooper C (2002b) Does a fracture at one site predict later fractures at other sites? A British cohort study. Osteoporosis International 13(8): 624–9.

Vestergaard P, Mosekilde L (2003) Fracture risk associated with smoking: a meta-analysis. Journal of Internal Medicine 254(6): 572.

Wakeman R, Shead PD, Jenner GH (2004) Ortho-geriatric liaison – the missing link. Journal of Bone and Joint Surgery 86B: 636–8.

Walker N, Norton R, Van der Hoorn S, Rodgers A et al. (1999) Mortality after hip fracture: regional variations in New Zealand. New Zealand Medical Journal 23(112): 269–71.

Walls AW, Steele JG, Sheiham A et al. (2000) Oral health and nutrition in older people. Journal of Public Health Dentistry 60(4): 304–7.

Wanless D (2002) Securing Our Future Health: Taking a long term view. Public Enquiry Unit, HM Treasury, London.

Ward D, Severs M, Dean T, Brooks N (2004) Care home versus hospital environments for rehabilitation of older people. (Cochrane Review). Cochrane Library, Issue 2.

Warner R (2000) The effectiveness of nursing in stroke units. Nursing Standard 14(25): 32–5.

Warwick D (2004) New concepts in orthopaedic thromboprophylaxis. Journal of Bone and Joint Surgery 86B(6): 788–92.

Watson K, Ranomhota S (2002) Preoperative fasting: we need a new consensus. Nursing Times 98: 15.

Webb G, Copeman J (1996) The Nutrition of Older Adults. Arnold, London.

Webster J (2002) Teamwork: understanding multi-professional working. Nursing Older People 14(3): 14–19.

Williams B, Grant G (1998) Defining 'person-centredness': making the implicit explicit. Health and Social Care in the Community 6(2): 84–94.

Willis S (1998) Falls in elderly people: is the risk suitably assessed? British Journal of Nursing 7(20): 1259–62.

Wilson L (2003) Continence and older people: the importance of functional assessment. Nursing Older People 15(4): 22–8.

Wittenberg R, Pickard L, Comas-Herrera A et al. (2001) Demand for long term care for older people in England to 2031. National Statistics Quarterly 12: 5–16.

Woolf AD, Akesson K (2003) Preventing fractures in elderly people. BMJ 327: 89–94.

Woolf AD, Pfleger B (2003) Burden of major musculoskeletal conditions. Bulletin of the World Health Organization, Geneva.

Wyld R, Nimmo W (1998) Do patients fasting before and after their operation receive their prescribed drug treatment? BMJ (Clinical Research Edition) 296: 6624.

Yeh SS, Schuster RW (1999) Geriatric cachexia: the role of cytokines. American Journal of Nutrition 70: 183-97.

Young J (1996) Caring for older people: rehabilitation and older people. BMJ 313: 677-81.

Young LJ, George J (2003) Do guidelines improve the process and outcomes of care in delirium? Age and Ageing 32: 525-8.

Zakriya K, Sieber FE, Christmas C, Wenz JF et al. (2004). Brief postoperative delirium in hip fracture patients affects functional outcome at three months. Anesthesia and Analgesia 98(6): 1798-1802.

Index